Journey
to
Gratitude

James P. Gills, MD

SILOAM

A JOURNEY TO GRATITUDE by James P. Gills, MD
Published by Siloam
Charisma Media/Charisma House Book Group
600 Rinehart Road
Lake Mary, Florida 32746

Greek definitions are derived from *Strong's Exhaustive Concordance of the Bible*, ed. James Strong, Nashville, TN: Thomas Nelson Publishers, 1997.

Visit the author's website at www.stlukeseye.com, DrJamesGills.com.

Library of Congress Cataloging-in-Publication Data

Names: Gills, James P., 1934- author.
Title: A journey to gratitude / by James P. Gills, MD.
Description: Lake Mary : Siloam, 2019. | Includes bibliographical
    references.
Identifiers: LCCN 2019024750 (print) | LCCN 2019024751 (ebook) | ISBN
    9781629996356 (trade paperback) | ISBN 9781629996363 (ebook)
Subjects: LCSH: God (Christianity)--Worship and love--Meditations. |
    Gratitude--Religious aspects--Christianity--Meditations.
Classification: LCC BV4817 .G55 2019 (print) | LCC BV4817 (ebook) |
DDC
    248.3--dc23
LC record available at https://lccn.loc.gov/2019024750
LC ebook record available at https://lccn.loc.gov/2019024751

Portions of this book were previously published by Creation House as *Exceeding Gratitude for the Creator's Plan*, ISBN 978-1-59979-155-5, copyright © 2007.

While the author has made every effort to provide accurate internet addresses at the time of publication, neither the publisher nor the author assumes any responsibility for errors or for changes that occur after publication. Further, the publisher does not have any control over and does not assume any responsibility for author or third-party websites or their content.

19 20 21 22 23 — 987654321
Printed in the United States of America

CONTENTS

Introduction vii

Day 1: The Transforming Power of Appreciation 1
Day 2: Radical Gratitude 4
Day 3: Discovering the Divine Designer 8
Day 4: Recognizing the Creator 12
Day 5: Anointed DNA 15
Day 6: Eternal DNA 18
Day 7: God the Father 21
Day 8: Revealed Through Christ 24
Day 9: Our Redeemer 27
Day 10: God the Holy Spirit 31
Day 11: A Divine Person 34
Day 12: The Word of God 37
Day 13: God's Word Revealed 40
Day 14: Divine Absolutes 43
Day 15: Love 46
Day 16: Salvation of Mankind 49
Day 17: Forgiveness 52
Day 18: Grace 56
Day 19: Guarding Our Faith 59
Day 20: Surrender to God 62
Day 21: Peace 65

Day 22: A Garden of Prayer............................ 68
Day 23: Divine Testing............................... 72
Day 24: Divine Destiny 75
Day 25: Divine Rest 78
Day 26: Divine Comfort.............................. 81
Day 27: Margin...................................... 85
Day 28: Healing 88
Day 29: Waiting on the Lord.......................... 91
Day 30: The Joy-Filled Life 95

Conclusion 99
Appendix: Nine Ways to Cultivate the Presence of
           God in Your Life 103
Notes... 109
About the Author 115

INTRODUCTION

I AM CONVINCED THAT the cause of much of life's unhappiness and many of life's failures is that we, as human beings, lack *exceeding gratitude* for our Creator. This faulty life perspective causes us to take His divine gift of life for granted. As a result, we live in discontent and misery, complaining about what we *don't* have and failing to express genuine appreciation for what we *do* have.

I am also convinced that by simply stopping to appreciate the world around us, as well as the marvelous *world* of life within us (i.e., our human body), our perspective of life can be transformed. This new perspective will reveal the Creator's redemptive plan and fill our hearts with exceeding gratitude for our Creator-Redeemer. This divine relationship will transform us into joyful, ennobled Christian steward-servants.

Our capacity for knowledge, without which we cannot appreciate life or the giver of life, must be understood as a special gift from our Creator. His grace—divine favor—bestowed upon mankind gives us the intelligence to pursue knowledge. Each individual must choose the source of knowledge to rely on for meaning in life. Your choice of worldview, philosophy, religion, or lack of religion will ultimately determine your level of appreciation for life as well as your destiny.

What is your worldview? Your life perspective? Where are you on the *appreciation scale*? Do you live in self-centered misery, or have you discovered the secret to personal destiny and deep satisfaction in life? Instead of suffering the effects of selfish unhappiness, you can learn to cultivate a lifestyle of radical gratitude by gaining knowledge of the wonders of life. This new perspective can be transforming as you learn to truly appreciate the divine gift of life you have been given.

The purpose of this book can be summed up in three key words:

1. *Appreciation* means to grasp the worth and value of something or someone, to esteem and properly revere them. God is Creator of the laws of nature; therefore, all of nature reveals God to us. Appreciation for the Creator's intelligent design deepens as we gain knowledge of the unfathomable generosity of our Creator-God.

2. *Adoration* is the spontaneous heart response to a revelation of our loving God and Savior, who desires intimate relationship with His highest creation—mankind. Adoration for our God fills us with praise and thanksgiving for His gift of life and brings us to repentance for our great sin of omission—our lack of appreciation in taking His gift of life for granted.

3. *Anointing* is the divine charisma of God, Himself, and it characterizes the beauty of a life lived in intimate relationship with God. As we learn to appreciate our Creator-Redeemer and ask Him to anoint our hearts and lives, we can rest in the joy and peace of Christ's redemption.

If you want to live a joy-filled life, you will need a change in perspective regarding the gift of life given to you. You will need to develop a profound appreciation for your Creator, who designed you before time began. Knowledge of this unfathomable design will birth appreciation within you. As you develop an attitude of exceeding gratitude for the Creator-Redeemer and His awesome gift of life, you will learn to live in satisfying, intimate relationship with Him.

The biblical truths of this devotional can bring a positive change to your life perspective. They can lead you into a deeper *appreciation* for the Creator, enable you to express sincere *adoration* to God, and teach you to live a satisfying, joy-filled, *anointed* life. Jesus promised: "I have come that they may have life, and that they may have it more abundantly" (John 10:10). May you become like a tree, "planted by the rivers of water" (Ps. 1:3). May you bask in the exquisite comfort of the "good shepherd" (John 10:11). And may your life blossom with the radiance of joy and peace that emanate from a heart filled with exceeding gratitude for the Creator's plan for the life He has given you to enjoy.

The Transforming Power of Appreciation

Knowledge of the creation reveals to us the nature of our Creator. As we behold the Creator's infinite hand in our universe, we begin to understand that He is outside of time or any other finite, limiting force. The Creator is eternal. And if He designed life with a divine purpose, it must be to unlock the secrets of eternity to our hearts. Jesus asked the Father to give eternal life to as many as He had given to the Son (John 17:2). He continued: "And this is eternal life, that they may know You, the only true God, and Jesus Christ whom You have sent" (v. 3). Learning to appreciate the Creator can be a beginning point for us to unlocking the eternal benefits of knowing God; receiving His Son, Jesus Christ; and thereby entering into eternal life.

Yet it has been my observation that even people of faith, born-again believers in Christ who love their Creator-Redeemer, seem to lack appreciation for His creation. They fail to comprehend the wondrous beauty all around them and may also abuse the gift of physical health the Creator has given them. Their lack of knowledge of the Creator's handiwork keeps them from fully appreciating the eternal benefits of life they have been given. Conversely you may have observed, with me, those people who have not surrendered to Christ as their Savior, who neverthe-less enjoy a deep appreciation for the wonders of creation. Their

1

scientific knowledge of the mysterious workings of life and the beauty of the laws of physics, for example, give them a wondrous perspective of life that evokes deep appreciation for the gift of life. It often sets them on a journey, as it did me, to surrender to the love of their Creator-Redeemer.

When these two realities—appreciation for creation and surrender to the Creator-Redeemer—unite in a person's heart, there is an explosion of hope, love, joy, purpose, and destiny. Only believers who learn to appreciate their Creator can truly enjoy the eternal benefits of the abundant life, which Jesus promised: "I have come that they may have life, and that they may have it more abundantly" (John 10:10). That new life perspective of deep appreciation in a believer's heart evokes adoration and worship of God. And this divine relationship in turn manifests the power of God's anointing in a life of worship, fulfilling our eternal destiny. It is this anointed life, restored to relationship with the Creator-Redeemer, that brings the deepest joy and satisfaction to the human heart. We never tire of reflecting on the wisdom of John Piper's maxim: "God is most glorified in me when I am most satisfied in Him."[1]

UNDERSTANDING APPRECIATION

What does it mean to truly appreciate? To be grateful? Webster's dictionary defines the terms for us. To *appreciate* is "to grasp the nature, worth, quality, or significance of; to value or admire highly; to judge with heightened perception or understanding: be fully aware of; to recognize with gratitude."[2] Similarly, the noun *appreciation* is defined as "a feeling or expression of admiration, approval, or gratitude; judgment, evaluation—especially: a favorable critical estimate; sensitive awareness—especially: recognition of aesthetic values."[3]

Grateful means "appreciative of benefits received."[4] To be grateful and fully appreciate the gift of life, we must acquire an increased awareness of its worth and a heightened perception of its significance. Appreciation involves placing such high value on something that it evokes our deep admiration. It also implies recognition of aesthetic values, which gain our unabashed approval and our expression of generous gratitude. It follows that to truly appreciate the *gift* of life, we must learn to appreciate the giver of life.

A lack of appreciation will inevitably cause us to take all of life for granted—not only ours but also the precious lives of those around us. I believe this faulty perspective of life is a sin of omission and is one of the greatest failures of mankind. When we truly appreciate our Creator, we will not take for granted the awesome gift of life He has given to us. For me, the personal discoveries of the gift of life, as seen through the microscope, caused an explosion of appreciation within my heart and mind for the Creator. Out of sheer gratitude for the unimaginable complexities of all cells, which form over two hundred different kinds of tissues in our body, my heart reached out to thank the One who made it all possible. In my humble acknowledgment of a Creator, I desired to know Him. And in seeking to know Him, I discovered Him, not only as my Creator but as my Redeemer as well.

PERSONAL REFLECTION

_____

_____

_____

Day 2

Radical Gratitude

T RUE APPRECIATION FOR God evokes the most profound expressions of gratitude, admiration, and worship of which the human spirit is capable. Ironically it is in those humble expressions of adoration to our Creator-Redeemer that we also find ultimate fulfillment and satisfaction in life.

Ellen Vaughn, in her book *Radical Gratitude*, recounts how the transcending power of a grateful heart caused men and women who faced hardship and tragedy to win in the face of life's overwhelming challenges. She cites the powerful views of gratitude that philosophers in the classical Western tradition have held.

> The Roman sage Cicero called gratitude not only the greatest of virtues but the parent of all others....Plato and Socrates wrote that citizens have a duty of obedience to the state based on gratitude for its benefits. Shakespeare wrote, "O Lord that lends me life, lend me a heart replete with thankfulness!" Immanuel Kant said that ingratitude was the "essence of vileness."[1]

The power of gratitude to impact our lives, according to the philosophers, lies in understanding that gratitude "is not only the greatest, but is the parent of all the other virtues."[2]

Conversely, all kinds of evil—the essence of vileness—gain entrance to our lives through the terrible vacuum in our hearts created by our lack of appreciation for our Creator. Every eternal virtue in life triumphs over evil when we learn to allow our hearts to be filled with gratitude. The apostle Paul confirmed the impact that expressing gratitude has on our lives.

> Rejoice in the Lord always. I will say it again: Rejoice!…Do not be anxious about anything, but in everything, by prayer and petition, with thanksgiving, present your requests to God. And the peace of God, which transcends all understanding, will guard your hearts and your minds in Christ Jesus.
>
> —Philippians 4:4, 6–7, niv

A personal relationship with God counteracts the destructive power of anxiety in our lives. The apostle Paul had his share of troubles, yet he declared confidently: "Who shall separate us from the love of Christ? Shall tribulation, or distress, or persecution, or famine, or nakedness, or peril, or sword?…Yet in all these things we are more than conquerors through Him who loved us" (Rom. 8:35, 37).

As we learn to place high value on the Creator and His creation, we discover the great value of our own lives as well as of the lives of others. This sense of significance in itself is a powerful impetus for overcoming life's challenges. Often our lack of appreciation can be heard in our whining complaints: "If only I had this" or "If only I could do that." These and similar statements reveal our selfish nature that lacks appreciation for God's divine gift of life to us. Instead of expressing gratitude daily for what we have, we focus on what we do not have. As a result, we are blinded to all of life's good things we could be enjoying.

Those are internal obstacles to seeing the beauty of life clearly. Our degree of spiritual sight hinges on the honesty and sincerity with which we appreciate our Lord. Many people do not appreciate the Lord and His gifts because they are content with the attractions of superficial observations and desires and they are selfish and proud. Answering the following question may be the beginning of a new life perspective for some: How can I remain indifferent to the marvelous design of my body and the Creator's eternal plans written within it?

Of course in acknowledging that we owe our lives to the Creator of life, we are expressing dependence on another, which is uncomfortable to our independent minds. However, if we admit the fact that we did not create ourselves, it follows that we cannot know the purpose for which we exist without consulting with the Creator. If we choose to go blindly through life without acknowledging our dependence on our Maker, we are doomed to live in the misery of ingratitude.

DIVINE DESTINY

I invite you to personally evaluate your level of appreciation for the gift of life and the giver of life as you continue to read this devotional. Knowing the satisfaction of discovering your eternal destiny—the divine purpose for which you were born—demands such an evaluation. Take the challenge to consider your lack of gratitude, first for the Creator and then for each aspect of the wondrous gift of life He has given you to enjoy. In such honest confrontation, you do not need to fear anything except the lack of appreciation that keeps you bound to failure in areas of your life. I encourage you to receive the promise

God made many years ago to His people, the Israelites, for the fulfillment of divine destiny: "I have set before you life and death, blessing and cursing; therefore *choose life, that both you and your descendants may live*" (Deut. 30:19, emphasis added).

PERSONAL REFLECTION

_____

_____

_____

_____

_____

_____

_____

_____

_____

_____

_____

_____

_____

Day 3

Discovering the Divine Designer

I F LIFE IS truly a gift from God and an expression of His grace and divine favor, then getting to know God must be the ultimate expression of human life. David Jeremiah describes grace as "the bridge over a chasm that seemed infinite—the canyon between our depravity and His holiness. That bridge is wide and sturdy and sure, beckoning us to cross over into a life too wonderful for us to imagine."[1]

Dr. Armand Nicholi, a Harvard professor, has taught a course for twenty-five years that compares the philosophical arguments of two of the most brilliant men of the twentieth century, Sigmund Freud and C. S. Lewis. Although the two men never met, Dr. Nicholi lays out their writings in his book as a way of allowing them to share their contrasting views on the profound topics of God, life, and love.[2] I encourage you to read Dr. Nicholi's book. The next several paragraphs are my attempt to recap some of his comparisons while expanding on them with a few of my personal observations.

Sigmund Freud, a devout atheist, and C. S. Lewis, an atheist-turned-believer, express polarizing views of the most fundamental issues of mankind that determine meaning in life. For example, on the question of the existence of God, "Freud asserts we possess intense, deep-seated wishes that form the basis for our concept of and belief in God." In our helplessness we seek protection; in our loneliness we seek companionship and comfort. Therefore, we "create" God in our image to meet our needs; He exists only in our minds as a fantasy of our wish fulfillment. Because we looked to our earthly father for protection in our childhood, most people exalt that idea and create a fantasy image of a divine Father to be our God. "Freud...advise[s] us to grow up and give up the 'fairy tales of religion.'"[3]

Lewis, in contrast to Freud's wish-fulfillment argument, stated that "the biblical worldview involves a great deal of despair and pain," which is certainly not to be wished for. To embrace the biblical worldview, one must first come to the understanding that he has violated the laws of morality and desperately needs forgiveness. The Christian worldview, according to Lewis, "begins to make sense only 'after you have realized that there is a real Moral Law, and a Power behind the law, and that you have broken that law and put yourself wrong with the Power.'" Lewis concluded that finding God begins in dismay rather than in comfort."[4]

Secondly, Lewis refutes the wishful-thinking argument of Freud on the basis that living in relationship with God also involves pain. Scripture teaches that we must submit our will to the will of God. Lewis notes that the process of "rendering back one's will, which we have so long claimed for our own, is, in itself, extraordinarily painful. To surrender a self-will inflamed and swollen with years of usurpation is a kind of death."[5]

Finally, Lewis reasons that "wishing for something [does] not rule out the existence of the object wished for—it may itself be evidence *for* its existence." We usually possess desires for things that exist. Lewis states, "'Creatures are not born with desires unless satisfaction for those desires exists...'" He then implies we all have a deep-seated desire, or wish, for a relationship with the Creator and for an existence beyond this life, though we often mistake it for something else."[6]

Lewis reasons: "If I find in myself a desire which no experience in this world can satisfy, the most probable explanation is that I was made for another world....If none of my earthly pleasures satisfy it, that does not prove that the universe is a fraud. Probably earthly pleasures were never meant to satisfy it, but only to arouse it, to suggest the real thing. If that is so, I must take care, on the one hand, never to despise, or be unthankful for, these earthly blessings, and on the other, never to mistake them for the something else of which they are only a kind of copy, or echo, or mirage.... *I must keep alive in myself the desire for my true country*, which I shall not find till after death....I must make it the main object of life to press on to that other country and to help others to do the same."[7] Lewis' purpose in life was expressed in those statements.

Freud recognized a similar unfulfilled desire in himself as that which Lewis defined. "In a paper published in 1899, Freud described a 'longing' that haunted him all of his life. This longing he associated with a desire to walk in the woods with his father, as he did as a child. He writes: 'I believe now that I was never free from a longing for the beautiful woods near our home, in which...I used to run off from my father, almost before I had learnt to walk.'"[8]

Lewis writes: "All your life an unattainable ecstasy has hovered just beyond the grasp of your consciousness. The day is coming when you will wake to find, beyond all hope, that you have attained it, or else, that it was within your reach and you have lost it forever."[9]

Thousands of years ago King Solomon, declared to be the wisest man who ever lived, warned: "Remember now your Creator in the days of your youth" (Eccles. 12:1). There is no other way to appreciate the gift of life you have been given. And in no other sphere can you hope to understand the divine purpose for which you have been created. The Old Testament prophet declared: "Have you not known? Have you not heard? The everlasting God, the LORD, the Creator of the ends of the earth, neither faints nor is weary. His understanding is unsearchable" (Isa. 40:28). Seeking to know this God is a life-time adventure that will unlock the mysteries of the wonderful gift of life you have been given.

Scripture teaches that everything that has been created had its origin in the bosom of the triune God—Father, Son, and Holy Ghost. Grasping this spiritual reality by faith will bring you into deeper worship and love for the One who formed you. And not only will seeking to know His purpose for your life bring fulfillment to you in your journey on earth; it will also reap great rewards for your future. According to Scripture, that future is forever—eternity spent with God, your Creator, your Father, your Savior.

As you observe creation in its beauty and appreciate the intricate details that point to a divine designer, you can discover many secrets about your Creator-God. And as you seek to know God as your Savior through Christ, the Son of God, the Holy Ghost will do His wonderful work of grace in your life. He will open your heart and mind to the truths of the Word of God.

PERSONAL REFLECTION

Day 4

Recognizing the Creator

T HE BIBLE TEACHES that God is the Creator of the heavens and the earth and all that is in them. From the first verse of the Bible to the last, it is clear that those "holy men of God," who "spoke as they were moved by the Holy Spirit" (2 Pet. 1:21) to write the Holy Scripture, accepted as fact the Creator. In the Book of Genesis we read the record of beginnings.

> In the beginning God created the heavens and the earth. The earth was without form, and void; and darkness was on the face of the deep. And the Spirit of God was hovering over the face of the waters.
>
> —GENESIS 1:1–2

We also read a lovely description of the beauty of the Earth God prepared for mankind.

> The LORD God planted a garden eastward in Eden, and there He put the man whom He had formed. And out of the ground the LORD God made every tree grow that is pleasant to the sight and good for food.
>
> —GENESIS 2:8–9

Our loving Creator gave us everything we see around us and provided us with exquisite senses—seeing, hearing, feeling, tasting, and smelling—to experience them to the full. He placed the first couple in a garden and gave them the assignment to cultivate and administrate it. They had all they needed to sustain life and to enjoy the presence of their Creator as He walked with them "in the cool of the day" (Gen. 3:8). And even after they disobeyed His command and lost fellowship with Him, creation did not lose all of its beauty and comfort.

DELIGHTING IN CREATION

Do you rush madly through the day, the month, the seasons of the year, scarcely noticing anything, except perhaps the inconvenience of a hot, humid summer day, pouring rain, or the bitterly cold wind of a December day? We have suggested that *gratitude* is the proper response to a God who has so abundantly blessed us with the multitudinous facets of nature. Our Creator not only made life possible but intended it to be enjoyable as well.

If you have not expressed appreciation for the creation of God that is all around you, why not start today? Ask the Holy Spirit to open your eyes to its wonders, its beauties, and the refreshing relaxation it holds for you. Begin to focus your senses on the natural phenomena you encounter every day. Touch the bark of a tree or the petals of a delicate flower, and allow yourself to marvel in the feeling. When you eat fresh fruit or vegetables, imagine them growing in their natural habitat, and be thankful. Behold the stars and planets in the night sky, and be thankful that you have the ability to do so.

The apostle Paul asserts that men everywhere are without excuse for not knowing God by observing the things He made.

> For since the creation of the world His invisible attributes are clearly seen, being understood by the things that are made, even His eternal power and Godhead, so that they are without excuse, because, although they knew God, they did not glorify Him as God, nor were thankful, but became futile in their thoughts, and their foolish hearts were darkened.
>
> —ROMANS 1:20–21

Paul explains that it is possible to know God's eternal power and His person by acknowledging the wonder of the creation around us and being thankful to Him for it. According to Scripture, there is a capacity in the human spirit to grasp the invisible attributes of God through the visible creation that He has made.

Of course we can, and must, get to know God more perfectly through relationship with His Son, Jesus Christ, who came to the earth to become our Savior. Yet we dare not ignore the wonderful opportunity He has given us to revel in the genius of the Creator—the Maker of heaven and earth.

PERSONAL REFLECTION

_____

_____

_____

_____

_____

Day 5

Anointed DNA

THERE IS A certain mystery surrounding the gift of life. We do not know precisely the way the soul is related to the body. We understand that the soul-spirit is the spiritual dimension of the person and the body is the physical dimension of the person. DNA is the template for the body, which is joined to the soul-spirit in God's own way. The brain is a physical organ of the body, and the mind is the intellectual expression of the soul. All are related integrally in God's design. We ask for the anointing of our DNA so that the beautiful, intricate unfolding of this comprehensive divine design is fulfilled in our lives.

It was the Creator's plan that our lives be the most beautiful expression of created life known to mankind. Our loving God created mankind to live in harmonious relationship with Him, which would be accompanied by His anointing on our unique expression of the dance of life. There is no instructor who can teach us this spiritual dance like the Word of God can. When we seek forgiveness of our sins and accept salvation through Christ, the Holy Spirit comes to dwell in our lives and give us a new nature. The Christian who is indwelled by the Holy Spirit is indwelled by God. And He begins His work to shed the love of God abroad in our hearts (Rom. 5:5). Then we begin to express the beauty of our spiritual lives through worship, prayer, and spontaneous rejoicing. We drop off the stoic, religious "person" in our lives who does not respond sincerely to the living God. And we become filled with spontaneous praise for His divine gift of life. As a result, our lives are characterized by intimate love, joy, peace, patience, kindness—all of the attributes of a loving Creator-God.

Life becomes a response of appreciation for everything God is, His creation, and His redemption of our lives—past, present, and future. This spiritual dance of life leads us into more intimate relationship with God through every season of our lives. As we progress to deeper and inexpressible adoration, we respond in complete surrender to the redemption of Christ and are reconciled to the will of our heavenly Father. Our dance of gratitude gives dignity to the human body, declaring that we are made according to a divine plan by a great God who loves us and cares only that we love Him in return.

This response to God affects our relationships with others as well. We begin to really care for people, even those who cause us trouble, by simply loving them. As we allow our grateful hearts to overcome all other obstacles, ours will become a godly love that cares for others more than ourselves. We become aware that our dance of life is not haphazard; it is ordered by God. As we meditate on the Word of God, we feel the presence of His Spirit within us orchestrating our spiritual dance. It may not often be a public expression of worship; it is most evident in a simple lifestyle that is surrendered to God.

Those who have sought God and found His precious anointing of their hearts, lives, and DNA guard themselves for their beloved, Christ alone. As they surrender their lives to Christ, He pours His love through them to others. Their lives are kept not for religion, but for relationship—intimate relationship with the Redeemer, Jesus Christ. And His life radiates through their smiles, words, attitudes, and actions.

Choosing to live a selfless life gives us a capacity to experience the love of God and His love for others. There are flowers that will close up their petals tightly when anything comes to cause pain and threaten their beautiful blooms. However, the selfless life does not reject even the pain of denying ourselves and taking up our cross, as Jesus taught us to do. (See Mark 8:34.) The anointed life does not have petals that close up in the face of difficulties and pain. We dare not become angry with God, rejecting Him when pain comes into our lives and despising His ways.

There are many ways to reject God, such as forsaking prayer and worship or neglecting to rejoice in the greatness of our God. When we lack purity, holiness, and a true appreciation of God, we are also rejecting Him. Even a lack of appreciation and respect for ourselves and for others causes us to reject the love of God for us. These grave errors always oppose our spiritual lives and hinder God's anointing from defining destiny in our lives.

To be recipients of His divine love, we must seek to know Him and call upon Him to anoint our lives by His Spirit. We live in the truth of our salvation, which is a fact of faith based conclusively on the premise "We love Him because He first loved us" (1 John 4:19). As we yield our lives to the business of loving God and doing our work in a godly way, we live in constant anticipation of His presence in our lives. It is that divine presence that we will enjoy throughout eternity.

PERSONAL REFLECTION

_____

_____

_____

_____

Day 6

Eternal DNA

W HILE WE CANNOT know for certain how the eternal expression of our lives in heaven will look, it is fascinating to consider our eternal response to God. In the same way that we are products of the DNA of our ancestors—all the way back to the first man formed by God from the dust of the earth—we are also made in the likeness of God, who is Spirit. Through our redemption in Christ, God Himself comes to dwell within our spirits, reconciling us to His love.

Because scientists have discovered such elaborate, divine orchestration of human life, beyond our imagination or understanding, it seems reasonable that some of the fundamental secrets of life locked into our natural DNA would have their spiritual counterparts in our eternal bodies. Admittedly, this is speculation. But we can point to the reality of our hope for the eternal bodies we will one day possess. (See 1 Corinthians 15.)

No matter how it occurs, we know that our "eternal DNA" will be beautiful. All God does is exquisite beyond our imagination, to such extraordinary heights that we are humbled by His majesty, beauty, wisdom, knowledge, and understanding. To think that this great God desires eternal relationship with each of us, calling us to be believers—walking in divine destiny—is unimaginable to our natural minds. Our "eternal DNA" is a future reality we can only thank God for creating, although we cannot imagine how it will be expressed throughout eternity.

Scripture teaches our marvelous potential for living a godly life.

> Grace and peace be multiplied to you in the knowl-
> edge of God and of Jesus our Lord, as His divine
> power has given to us all things that pertain to life
> and godliness, through the knowledge of Him who
> called us by glory and virtue, by which have been
> given to us exceedingly great and precious prom-
> ises, that through these you may be partakers of the
> divine nature.
>
> —2 PETER 1:2–4

Redemptive characteristics, such as being "partakers of the divine nature," reveal the unfathomable results of enhancing the life, design, and function of your DNA. These promises are actively at work in your life to enable you to enjoy an intimate relationship with your Creator. You will be filled with grace, favor, and peace when your unique individuality is conformed to the image of Christ. (See Romans 8:29.) In this anointed way of life the beautiful character of Christ—His love, grace, peace, and joy—will flow through you to others.

God is love, and the more you seek Him, allowing the Holy Spirit to work in your heart, the greater your spiritual response of love becomes. Because God is love (1 John 4:7) and you are made in the image of God (Gen. 1:26), God's love is the only true source of satisfaction for your heart. Your highest response to the Creator's eternal plan for your life is to bow before Him in humble *adoration* for creating in you a capacity to live in relation-ship with Him. Webster's Dictionary defines the verb *adore* as "to worship or honor as a deity or as divine; to regard with loving admiration and devotion."[1]

Do you readily identify with intense affection inherent in

adoration? Reverent admiration? Devotion? Gifts pale in comparison with the treasure of the person worthy of our adoration. What the giver does is insignificant in light of who He is. To be with Him is the ultimate pleasure and satisfaction. To please Him is your delight and deep desire.

If you have experienced the rescue of your soul by Christ, your divine Redeemer, there will be a natural (or supernatural) response to your new "owner"—inexpressible gratitude, devotion, and expressed adoration. Not content to just receive the gifts Christ gives us, we simply want to be with Him, to enjoy the nearness of His presence. That is the essence of adoration—to experience the spiritual purpose for which our bodies and DNA are joined to our soul, we must acknowledge our Creator as the giver of life as well as the Redeemer of our souls. This is the spiritual expression of our DNA. Without Him there is no dance of life, no hope, no joy, no fulfillment—only a dirge of grief, pain, loneliness, and ultimate death.

We decide whether we will adore our Maker. The weight of that choice is amazing to me. That choice—to adore the Creator-Redeemer—is the most important issue of life. Other choices are important, but this is the basic issue that will determine the expression of our DNA and our destiny. It is not enough to give intellectual assent in acknowledging a Creator. Only in cultivating an adoring relationship with our Redeemer can we experience the ultimate satisfaction our Creator ordained for our lives—for eternity.

PERSONAL REFLECTION

Day 7

GOD THE FATHER

PERHAPS ONE OF the most awesome experiences for a man or woman is to hold his or her firstborn infant, the fruit of the person's union, in his or her arms. Scientists have been fascinated with the study of human genetics for many decades. The wonder of a female ovum uniting with a male sperm to create a human life is an awesome reality indeed.

Lee Strobel, a journalist and former atheist, set out on a quest for scientific proof of Darwinian evolution, interviewing leading scientists of our day. He interviewed Jonathan Wells, a holder of two PhDs, one in molecular and cell biology from Berkeley. He later worked as a postdoctoral research biologist at Berkeley. Strobel asked him, "Let's say a scientist someday actually manages to produce amino acids from a realistic atmosphere of the early earth.... How far would that be from creating a living cell?" Dr. Wells responded, "Oh, *very* far. *Incredibly* far... You would have to get the right number of the right kinds of amino acids to link up to create a protein molecule—and that would still be a long way from a living cell. Then you'd need dozens of protein molecules, again in the right sequence, to create a living cell. The odds against this are astonishing. The gap between nonliving chemicals and even the most primitive living organism is absolutely tremendous."[1]

Dr. Wells continued, speaking authoritatively, "You can't make a living cell. There's not even any point in trying. It would

21

be like a physicist doing an experiment to see if he can get a rock to fall upwards all the way to the moon....In other words, if you want to create life, on top of the challenge of somehow generating the cellular components out of nonliving chemicals, you would have an even bigger problem in trying to put the ingredients together in the right way....The problem of assembling the right parts in the right way at the right time and at the right place, while keeping out the wrong material, is simply insurmountable."[2]

"OUR FATHER"

Strobel also questioned former Texas A&M professor Walter Bradley, coauthor of *The Mystery of Life's Origin*. Bradley demonstrated that none of "the various theories advanced by scientists for how the first living cell could have been naturalistically generated—including random chance, chemical affinity, self-ordering tendencies, seeding from space, deep-sea ocean vents, and using clay to encourage prebiotic chemicals to assemble...can withstand scientific scrutiny."[3]

Bradley shares the view of many scientists that the "difficulties in bridging the yawning gap between nonlife and life mean that there may very well be no potential of ever finding a theory for how life could have arisen spontaneously. That's why he's convinced that the 'absolutely overwhelming evidence' points toward an intelligence behind life's creation." Bradley further stated, "I think people who believe that life emerged naturalistically need to have a great deal more faith than people who reasonably infer that there's an Intelligent Designer."[4]

The real question becomes, On what purpose is this intelligent design predicated? How can we discern the mysterious beauty of the designer? The answer lies in the divine revelation to our spirit of the Creator Himself—our Father. Even Nobel Prize–winning biochemist Francis Crick, who discovered the molecular structure of DNA, ascribed the word *miracle* to the origin of life. "An honest man, armed with all the knowledge available to us now, could only state that in some sense, the origin of life appears at the moment to be almost a miracle, so many are the conditions which would have had to have been satisfied to get it going."[5]

What could be the purpose of this miracle? What is the intelligent designer's motive for creating such exquisitely complex life on a planet of apparent insignificance in the limitless scope of the universe?

It is God's very nature to be a Father. He delighted to express that divine nature in creation. Who can fathom the love of God that created mankind because He wanted to express His divine love to them—to relate to them as His children? Our gratitude for the gift of life will be inspired primarily as we experience personal relationship with the giver of all life—God the Father.

PERSONAL REFLECTION

_____

_____

_____

_____

_____

_____

_____

Day 8

REVEALED THROUGH CHRIST

J ESUS, THE SON of God, came to the earth to reveal the Father to us. He spoke often of His Father and prayed to Him. And Jesus taught His disciples to begin their prayer by addressing the Father: "Our Father in heaven, Hallowed be Your name" (Matt. 6:9).

According to Scripture, no one on earth has seen God the Father. It is true that Moses cried out to see the glory of God. God granted his desire, made a place for him to hide, and then allowed His great goodness to pass by him. (See Exod. 33:19.) That glimpse of God transformed Moses and caused His face to shine so brightly that he had to cover it with a veil because the children of Israel could not look upon it.

Yet the New Testament scriptures plainly declare, "No one has seen God at any time. The only begotten Son, who is in the bosom of the Father, He has declared Him" (John 1:18). And when Philip, Jesus' disciple, asked Him to show them the Father, Jesus answered Him.

> Have I been with you so long, and yet you have not known Me, Philip? He who has seen Me has seen the Father; so how can you say, 'Show us the Father'? Do you not believe that I am in the Father, and the Father in Me?
>
> —JOHN 14:9–10

It was John who described the eternal essence of Christ so vividly for us: "And the Word became flesh and dwelt among us, and we beheld His glory, the glory as of the only begotten of the Father, full of grace and truth" (John 1:14). Jesus showed us the character of our heavenly Father, reflected in the phrase "full of grace and truth." Yet even Old Testament saints such as the prophet Isaiah understood that God was a Father to them.

> Doubtless You are our Father, though Abraham was ignorant of us, and Israel does not acknowledge us. You, O LORD, are our Father; our Redeemer from Everlasting is Your name.
>
> —ISAIAH 63:16

ETERNAL LOVE

Because the first couple, Adam and Eve, chose to disobey God and walk independently from Him, God sacrificially sought to redeem mankind from sin so that those who seek relationship with Him could enjoy the Father's love.

So through Christ's sacrifice on Calvary, God restored the possibility for any man or woman to be redeemed from sin and reconciled to relationship with God as their Father. Our eternal Father offers His loving care, protection, provision, purpose, and much more to all who call Him Father. As we are reconciled to our heavenly Father through accepting the sacrifice of His Son for our sins, we can look forward to living and reigning with Him eternally in His wonderful kingdom.

One of the most endearing portraits of our loving heavenly Father was painted by Jesus in His parable that we call "the prodigal son." The youngest of his father's two sons, this "prodigal" asked for his inheritance before the customary time and then left the father's house and went to a "far country" where he "wasted his possessions with prodigal living" (Luke 15:13). Then there arose a famine in the land, and the boy had nothing to eat. This young man, once accustomed to fine living, got a job feeding pigs, and he was so hungry that he longed to eat the "pods that the swine ate" (v. 16). Then he "came to himself" (v. 17) and began to consider the abundance of his father's house, where even the servants had plenty to eat. Filled with remorse, he decided to return home and repent to his father, saying, "I have sinned against heaven and before you" (v. 18). He reasoned that he could ask to be made a hired servant and at least escape hunger.

Yet we know from Luke 15:20–24 that the forgiving love that runs toward a repentant prodigal is what we can expect from our heavenly Father when we make one step toward Him. His loving heart restores us to our position in the family of God that mankind lost in the fall through waywardness. It is an unfathomable source of gratitude to consider that God Himself loves all of humanity with such intense desire to do good for us, in spite of our failures. As you meditate on the love of God the Father, be quick to express your love and praise to Him. He will enlarge your capacity to know Him and to sense His presence and purpose in your life. And He will forgive any wrongs you have done in life. Such love causes us to bow in adoration before our God, declaring, "Our Father in heaven, hallowed be Thy name."

PERSONAL REFLECTION

Day 9

Our Redeemer

T HOUGH THE DISCIPLES failed Jesus in His hour of agony, they became recipients of His wonderful redemption after Jesus' resurrection. And tradition tells us that most of them, as the founders of the church Jesus died for, died as martyrs because of their devotion to the Lord. Some of the disciples gave us the New Testament scriptures, and all were empowered by the Holy Spirit to preach the gospel to a pagan world. Years later an aged John wrote about this:

> That which was from the beginning, which we have heard, which we have seen with our eyes, which we have looked upon, and our hands have handled, concerning the Word of life—the life was manifested, and we have seen, and bear witness, and declare to you that eternal life which was with the Father and was manifested to us.
>
> —1 John 1:1–2

The lives of these apostles were transformed because they had touched the Christ, who was full of grace and truth. And our lives can undergo this same transformation, as millions who have already received the wonderful grace and truth of Christ's salvation can testify.

Jesus knew that He would suffer many things, and he

27

prepared His disciples for it. He told them He would be rejected by religious leaders, be killed, and rise again after three days. (See Mark 8:31.) But His disciples could not stand the thought of His death, and on one occasion Peter even rebuked the Christ for speaking of it (Mark 8:32), which in turn brought him a stern rebuke from the Lord.

As Eric L. Knick put it,

> John the Baptist was baptizing in the river Jordan, when he looked up one day and saw Jesus coming toward him. He declared: "Behold! The Lamb of God who takes away the sin of the world!" (John 1:29). Through His death on the cross, Christ fulfilled every Old Testament "type" of the justice for mankind's sin required by a holy God. Jesus Christ became the spotless Lamb of God. A blood sacrifice was required to atone for sin. And the Book of Hebrews tells us that the blood of bulls and goats was not enough to provide a complete remedy for sin (see Heb. 9:13–14). That would require the death of the sinless Son of God.[1]

Knick went on to write,

> Our humanistic culture declares: "There are many ways to God. It is not important what you believe or in whom, but only *that* you believe." To that errant philosophy Scripture responds powerfully, declaring redemption through Christ alone: "Nor is there salvation in any other, for there is no other name under heaven given among men by which we must be saved" (Acts 4:12).[2]

THE RISEN MESSIAH

Only through the death of Christ could He fulfill His divine mission as the Messiah, the anointed One, sent to redeem all of mankind from the darkness and death of sin. Yet if He had not been raised from the dead, all of His suffering would have been in vain. The apostle Paul explains:

> If in this life only we have hope in Christ, we are of all men the most pitiable. But now Christ is risen from the dead, and has become the firstfruits of those who have fallen asleep. For since by man came death, by Man also came the resurrection of the dead. For as in Adam all die, even so in Christ all shall be made alive.
>
> —1 CORINTHIANS 15:19–22

Historians declare that there is more evidence of the resurrection of our Lord, Jesus Christ, than of any other event in antiquity. Through the resurrection of Christ we have hope of eternal life with God. Death, which entered through sin (death was not God's design for Adam), was overcome through Christ so that we could be raised from death to live with Him forever. Scripture is full of comfort for believers, teaching us that we will be given a glorified body to live in heaven with God and with all the saints who have gone on before.

We conclude our brief look at the wonderful Son of God, who became our resurrected Lord, by pausing to appreciate the wonder and love revealed in the Scripture verse most often quoted:

For God so loved the world that He gave His only

begotten Son, that whoever believes in Him should
not perish but have everlasting life.

—JOHN 3:16

Gratitude and joy flood the heart as we ask Him to redeem
us from our sin. Christ forgives, cleanses, heals, and delivers
the seeking soul from the destructive power of sin and gives us
eternal life.

PERSONAL REFLECTION

_____

_____

_____

_____

_____

_____

_____

_____

_____

_____

_____

Day 10
God the Holy Spirit

T HEOLOGIANS REFER TO God the Holy Spirit as the third person of the Trinity. While we must be careful not to err in separating God into three distinct gods for our discussion of the Holy Spirit, it will be helpful to focus on His *function* as God. According to Scripture, the Spirit of God was present in creation: "In the beginning God created the heavens and the earth. The earth was without form, and void; and darkness was on the face of the deep. And the Spirit of God was hovering over the face of the waters" (Gen. 1:1–2). When God spoke, "Let there be light" (v. 3), it seems that it was the Spirit of God who "performed it."

God Is Spirit

Jesus declared to the woman at the well: "God is Spirit, and those who worship Him must worship in spirit and truth" (John 4:24). So while we discuss the Holy Spirit as a part of the Trinity, and endeavor to learn how to relate to Him in a biblical way, we need to understand that God *is* Spirit. Again, we are confronted with the reality of the transcendent, divine mystery of the Trinity—a triune Godhead.

When God decided to create mankind, He said: "Let Us make man in Our image, according to Our likeness" (Gen. 1:26). Scripture acknowledges both a plurality in the Godhead—"Let Us"—and a consensus of purpose among them. To be created in the image of God, who is Spirit, necessarily implies that we are in essence spiritual beings. That is to say, we are more than a biological phenomenon made of chemicals. The apostle Paul referred to this reality when he prayed.

> Now may the God of peace Himself sanctify you completely; and may your whole *spirit, soul,* and *body* be preserved blameless at the coming of our Lord Jesus Christ.
> —1 THESSALONIANS 5:23, EMPHASIS ADDED

Though this spiritual side of human life has been neglected by many and is completely rejected by naturalists and secularists, it is taught throughout Scripture as an eternal reality. Accepting this biblical truth will determine much of your worldview. The Genesis account of the origin of mankind is simple.

> And the LORD God formed man of the dust of the ground, and breathed into his nostrils the breath of life; and man became a living being.
> —GENESIS 2:7

In light of the awesome scientific data we are discussing regarding the complexity of our unique DNA and the cellular structure of our bodies, the simplicity of this description of mankind's creation is striking. God formed man from the dust of the ground and breathed His breath of life into him. Scientists now know that our bodies are indeed composed of the same elements that form the dust of the earth. Yet the structure of every microscopic cell of the human body is incredible in its form and function.

After God formed man, He breathed life into his nostrils. As we mentioned, Scripture declares that God is Spirit. (See John

4:24.) The Hebrew word translated *spirit* in Genesis chapter 1 is *ruwach*, which is also translated as "wind" or "breath." Another Hebrew word, *neshamah*, is used to describe God breathing His breath into the first man's body, who "became a living being" (Gen. 2:7). *Neshamah* can be translated as "wind, vital breath, divine inspiration, and intellect." From this biblical account of the creation of mankind, which shows mankind receiving the breath of life from the Spirit of God, we can conclude that the essence of mankind's life is *spiritual*.

As an ophthalmologist, I see a lot of people who are nearsighted, which means they only see the things that are up close. All of us can be considered nearsighted spiritually when we fail to see the overall view of God's purpose for creating mankind. We focus too often on our personal plans and desires, failing even to consider the concerns of those around us whom we love. Many times we are not aware of God's desire for us.

The apostle James describes the brevity of our lives: "Why, you do not even know what will happen tomorrow. What is your life? You are a mist that appears for a little while and then vanishes" (James 4:14, NIV). In the grand scheme of things, our lives seem insignificant. Only as we focus on God with the help of the Holy Spirit can we begin to appreciate the eternal realities of life. When we believe in His promises, our focus is no longer shortsighted and placed on the things of this world. We see the distant view—eternity, the greatness of all reality. This is when we begin to comprehend who God really is.

PERSONAL REFLECTION

_____

_____

_____

Day 11

A DIVINE PERSON

THE HOLY SPIRIT is perhaps the most misunderstood member of the Godhead. Maybe because we have difficulty relating to God as Spirit and can more easily identify with the natural relationships of a father and son. Many tend to regard the Holy Spirit as an influence, a force, or another intangible being. However, the Holy Spirit is revealed in Scripture as a divine personality.

Perhaps considering other names given to the Holy Spirit in Scripture will help us to understand Him better. In the Gospel of John, He is called the Comforter, which can also be translated "Counselor, Helper, Advocate, Intercessor, Strengthener, and Standby." (See John 16:7, AMP.) Jesus declared the Holy Spirit to be the "Spirit of truth" (John 14:17) and the Helper who teaches. (See John 14:26, NASB.) The New Testament epistles confirm these wonderful facets of the work of the Holy Spirit in the lives of believers.

THE WORK OF THE HOLY SPIRIT

What a wonder it is that the Holy Spirit can be entreated to reveal the love of God to our hearts and to do His precious, divine work in our lives. Jesus made it clear in Luke 11:11–13 that our heavenly Father wants to give us the Holy Spirit.

Jesus declared that when He ascended into heaven to the Father, He would send the Holy Spirit to do His divine work in the earth. He then described the work of the Holy Spirit on earth. (See John 16:8–11.)

It is the work of the Holy Spirit to convict our hearts first and then show us our need of a Savior. Then He teaches us and gives us wisdom for life, revealing our purpose and destiny that God intended for us. It is His divine unction that transforms us and enables us to do the will of God. He gives us divine abilities (gifts of the Holy Spirit) to empower us to fulfill our divine destiny.

THE FRUIT OF THE HOLY SPIRIT

As we mentioned, we are dependent on the precious Holy Spirit to show us that we are sinners in need of a Savior and then guide us into the truth of righteous living in every area of our lives. We need Him to give us power over the evil one, the devil, who was defeated through Christ's death on Calvary. To grow in our faith, the New Testament epistles admonish believers to "walk in the Spirit" (Gal. 5:16), to "live in the Spirit" (Gal. 5:25), and to "be filled with the Spirit" (Eph. 5:18). And the apostle Paul declares plainly that believers are the temples of the Holy Spirit, who indwells us (1 Cor. 3:16). What will our lives look like if we live and walk in the Spirit? Scripture describes the beauty of such a life.

> But the fruit of the Spirit is love, joy, peace, longsuf-
> fering, kindness, goodness, faithfulness, gentleness,
> self-control. Against such there is no law....If we live
> in the Spirit, let us also walk in the Spirit.
> —GALATIANS 5:22–23, 25

Carefully consider this list of the fruit of the Spirit to deter-mine how much your life looks like it. Learning to yield to the

Holy Spirit in every situation of life will cause you to grow in grace, displaying a godly character filled with love, joy, peace, longsuffering, kindness, goodness, faithfulness, gentleness, and self-control. While none of us can produce such godly qualities all by ourselves, we can trust the Holy Spirit to fill us with the love of God and live His life through us. The apostle Paul declared, "The love of God has been poured out in our hearts by the Holy Spirit who was given to us" (Rom. 5:5).

THE ANOINTING OF THE HOLY SPIRIT

The work of God in all ages has been attributed to the Spirit of God. Christ Himself accomplished His work on earth by the anointing of the Holy Spirit.

As we bow our hearts in humble gratitude for the gift of the Holy Spirit, He will accomplish His divine work in our lives. He will give to us the things of Jesus (John 16:14), help us to pray (Rom. 8:26), transform us (2 Cor. 3:18), and fill us with the love of God (Rom. 5:5). To be filled with the Spirit means to be yielded to Him, obeying Him as He changes us into the image of Christ. This is what the kingdom of God is all about: "righteousness and peace and joy in the Holy Spirit" (Rom. 14:17). When the Holy Spirit is present in our lives, we must remember that He is not the resident—He is the president. As He mediates the presence of God to us, our minds and souls are opened so that it seems as if we are standing in the very courts of heaven.

PERSONAL REFLECTION

_____

_____

_____

DAY 12
THE WORD OF GOD

T HE BIBLICAL ACCOUNT of the beginnings of our world simply declares, "Then God *said*, 'Let there be…' and there was" (Gen. 1:3, emphasis added). According to Scripture, God created everything we see through the omnipotent power of His word. And the New Testament declares that He *upholds* everything by the power of His word. (See Hebrews 1:3.)

We understand that the *written* Word of God comprises the Old and New Testaments of the Bible. It was recorded when "holy men of God spoke as they were moved by the Holy Spirit" (2 Pet. 1:21). Scripture teaches that the *living* Word is Jesus Christ. Jesus declared that He is the living bread that came down from heaven. (See John 6:51.) He explained, "The words that I speak to you are spirit, and they are life" (John 6:63). He is God incarnate, who was made flesh and dwelled among us. (See John 1.) As we embrace the divine mystery of the eternal truths written in the Word of God, we understand they cannot exist apart from Christ, the living Word of God. It is precisely this mystery, the exquisite blending of fragrances of every aspect of divinity in creation, that evokes awe, deep worship, and appreciation for our Maker.

Pursuing God by studying His Word is one of the greatest pursuits in life. If we hope to know the God of the Bible, it is vital that we read the Word of God from beginning to end, not once, but many times. Continual study of Scripture will produce great benefits, planting living truth into our hearts and minds and enabling us to fulfill our eternal purpose in life. Men of great faith such as John Wesley, George Whitfield, and others loved the Word of God. And these men were used mightily by God to bring great revivals and transformations of their societies. It was their insatiable pursuit of God through His Word that made them great worshippers of God as well.

THE LAW OF GOD

Even Old Testament saints learned to know God and to love and obey Him through surrendering in obedience to His law. The psalmist understood the omnipotent power contained in the law of God.

> The law of the LORD is perfect, converting the soul; the testimony of the LORD is sure, making wise the simple; the statutes of the LORD are right, rejoicing the heart; the commandment of the LORD is pure, enlightening the eyes; the fear of the LORD is clean, enduring forever; the judgments of the LORD are true and righteous altogether.
>
> —PSALM 19:7–9

Have you ever received a birthday card that said just the words of love you wanted to hear and made you want to cry with gratitude and joy? That card was written by someone unknown to you. But it was purchased by someone who loves you and wants to express that love to you. The Bible is like that. It is God's love letter to you, uniquely applied to your life situation. As you seek the Holy Spirit to quicken the Word of God to your mind and heart, you will have the sense that though the

Bible was written long ago, it is still applicable to your personal situation right now. God is speaking through it to you—out of the love of His heart.

The psalmist also expressed an insatiable love for the Torah—the Law of God. He declared: "The law of Your mouth is better to me than thousands of coins of gold and silver....Oh, how I love Your law! It is my meditation all the day" (Ps. 119:72, 97). If you feel as if the Bible is just words on a page, I encourage you to begin to pray: *Lord, this is Your Word. Please help me to love it and meditate on its truths and apply it to my life.*

The Word of God itself will produce awe and reverence in the serious student. Again, the psalmist declared: "Let all the earth fear the LORD; let all the inhabitants of the world stand in awe of Him" (Ps. 33:8). As you meditate on its eternal truths, ask the Holy Spirit to make them a reality in your life. The more you meditate on the wonder of your Creator and the beauty of His creation, the more you will begin to appreciate the omnipotence of your sovereign God.

PERSONAL REFLECTION

_____

_____

_____

_____

_____

_____

Day 13
God's Word Revealed

G OD FIRST REVEALED the omnipotent power of His word
when He spoke the universe into existence in creation.
And His voice continued speaking to His highest creation—
mankind. The first couple, Adam and Eve, heard His voice
in the cool of the day in that beautiful garden where He had
placed them. Even after they disobeyed His voice and brought
calamity on the entire human race, He came to them.

The patriarchs—Abraham, Isaac, and Jacob, as well as Noah,
Moses, Joshua, and others, had dramatic encounters with the
voice of God. They understood the power of His word to them
in that they obeyed it and received divine promises. To the
Old Testament prophets, priests, and kings, God continued
speaking His word to guide the course of humanity. In His
pursuit of them, in His divine love—as God is love—He continued to reveal Himself through His word to His people.

The Bible is self-vindicating in its declaration that "prophecy
never came by the will of man, but holy men of God spoke as
they were moved by the Holy Spirit" (2 Pet. 1:21). Of course
there were long periods of time when, because of mankind's
rejection of the word of God, the Scriptures lament: "The word
of the LORD was rare in those days; there was no widespread
revelation" (1 Sam. 3:1). And there were the terribly dark four
hundred years between the close of the Old Testament era

and the New Testament Gospels, during which there seems to have been complete silence from God.

CHRIST, THE WORD

Breaking that desperate, dark silence of hundreds of years after the Old Testament prophets ceased speaking must have made the words of John's Gospel exquisitely beautiful to the hearers of his day. He described Jesus as the incarnate Word of God in his opening sentences.

Yet how can we ever comprehend the Word as a divine person? How can we really fathom the infinitely divine when we are so finite? Until we pursue that divine mystery, we cannot appreciate, admire, and esteem the Word—the written Word or the Christ—as we should. Years later John was given a vision of the eternally reigning Christ as the Word of God, as described in the Book of Revelation.

When we behold Christ as the King of kings, our sovereign Lord, it is difficult to imagine the humility that accompanied His incarnation. Yet the Word of God had to become man, humbling Himself to become a servant of men to redeem mankind and then be exalted to His rightful place as Lord of all. The apostle Paul explains this humbling of divinity.

> Let this mind be in you which was also in Christ Jesus, who, being in the form of God, did not consider it robbery to be equal with God, but made Himself of no reputation, taking the form of a bondservant, and coming in the likeness of men. And being found in appearance as a man, He humbled Himself and became obedient to the point of death, even the death of the cross. Therefore God

also has highly exalted Him and given Him the
name which is above every name, that at the name
of Jesus every knee should bow, of those in heaven,
and of those on earth, and of those under the earth,
and that every tongue should confess that Jesus
Christ is Lord, to the glory of God the Father.

—PHILIPPIANS 2:5–11

Jesus taught us how to live humbly in right relationship to the
Word of God. He declared that He was completely dependent
on the words of His Father, doing nothing that He did not hear
from His Father: "I am able to do nothing from Myself [indepen-
dently, of My own accord—but only as I am taught by God and
as I get His orders]" (John 5:30, AMPC). Filled with the Spirit of
God, Christ fulfilled His divine destiny, walking in complete obedience to the Father's will.

Scripture teaches that "the Word of God is living and powerful, and sharper than any two-edged sword, piercing even to
the division of soul and spirit, and of joints and marrow, and is
a discerner of the thoughts and intents of the heart" (Heb. 4:12).
And the apostle Paul instructs us how to wage war against the
enemies of our souls, using the "sword of the Spirit, which is the
word of God" (Eph. 6:17). As the written Word fills our minds
and hearts with illumination—spiritual understanding—by the
power of the Holy Spirit, we can truly know Christ, the living
Word, and grow in grace in our personal relationship with Him.

PERSONAL REFLECTION

_____

_____

_____

Day 14
Divine Absolutes

The Creator of all gave us a comprehensive designer's manual, in which He clearly indicates how we are to think and then act in every situation in life. The Word of God delineates His divine principles to us. These divine principles for life should be considered absolute truth because the Maker of all things has hardwired the necessary constraints they imply into us for our well-being.

When Moses was used by God to deliver over two million Israelites from the misery of slavery under the oppressive rule of Pharaoh in Egypt, this great multitude of people began moving toward the Promised Land, leaving behind all that had been familiar to them for over four hundred years. It was absolutely necessary that they be governed by specific social restraints to prevent potential chaos. So God gave Moses the laws and social ordinances that would order the lives of the Israelites in every situation they faced as a nation.

The Ten Commandments are still relevant to society today, and they are responsible for much of the peace, tranquility, and order we enjoy as Americans. Many of the divine principles they teach, especially regarding human dignity and respect for others, are embedded in the rule of law established by our national Constitution.

These commandments of God cannot be broken without grave consequences, both to the human psyche and to society.

Yet in His mercy God knew that mankind was helpless to keep His Law because of the power of sin that had entered the world. So He prescribed a system of sacrifices to teach them of the need for atonement for their sins. Through this means those who sincerely wanted to obey God but failed could repent and offer a blood sacrifice. This would result in their sins being covered.

It is in that context that Christ came to earth to become the spotless "Lamb of God" (John 1:29) and shed His blood as a supreme sacrifice for the sins of the whole world. He made it possible for us to be restored to right relationship with God. His sacrifice for sin also made it possible for us to become obedient children of God, filled with the blessings of God.

The blessing of obeying the commandments of God is not limited to the benefits of the social order they provide. The wonderful power of keeping God's commandments is reflected in communion with God that we enjoy through obedience as well.

It was very clear from the time Moses received the Commandments on the mount that God intended for the people to obey them. And these laws were never to be rejected, substituted, or replaced by future generations with different values and mindsets. On the contrary, Scripture teaches clearly that they were to be taught very carefully to succeeding generations (Deut. 6:6–7).

These instructions were followed by warnings not to forget the Lord and serve other gods, "lest the anger of the LORD your God be aroused against you and destroy you from the face of the earth" (Deut. 6:15). Of course the history of the nation of Israel records not only the blessings of their obedience but also the consequences of their disobedience.

The Law of Love

There are those who believe that because we are living during the centuries following the death of Christ, we are not subject to the Law of God. They conclude that we are living under *grace* now, since Christ died for our sins. However, Christ Himself taught that He did not come to do away with the law but to fulfill it (Matt. 5:17).

Of course the entire New Testament confirms the reality of walking in the redemption of God through expressing our gratitude by obedience to His commandments. Yet it is not an obedience of duty that is required but a relationship of love. And we do not obey in order to be saved from our sin but out of love because we have received His great grace that has forgiven our sin. Out of love for our Redeemer we pursue an intimate relationship with our Creator and Savior that is absolutely satisfying. This divine relationship motivates us to love our neighbor, which Jesus defined as anyone we see in need and wounded along the road of life. (See Luke 10:25–37.) As we truly fall in love with Christ, we will say with the psalmist, "I delight to do Your will, O my God, and Your law is within my heart" (Ps. 40:8).

PERSONAL REFLECTION

_____

_____

_____

_____

Day 15

Love

L OVE—THAT POWERFUL FOUR-LETTER word that is perhaps one of the most misused and misunderstood words in the human language—haunts, tantalizes, fills with hope, dashes to despair, and creates the greatest pursuit in all of life. In the final analysis love eludes the hearts and minds of many, leaving them feeling unloved and alone in life. At least, their *concept* of love has not been fulfilled, which causes them to suffer feelings of discontent and an ache of unbearable emptiness. They fail to find satisfaction despite their mad pursuit of the thing they call love.

It is perplexing for a person without Christ to find love so elusive. Listen to any hit song from the latest brokenhearted pop recording artist, and you will hear the pain inflicted through broken promises of love. Yet this emotional pain is not limited to failed adult romance; it stalks children, the elderly, and everyone who experiences circumstances that make them feel alone and unloved.

Where does one go to find the love that will satisfy the deepest yearnings of the human heart? Are those desires even legitimate, or are they selfish? Why do some people seem to "have it all together" and others feel neglected and lonely, even though they enter into relationships of marriage, parenting, community and church activities, friendship, and employment? These are just a few of the questions people ask relating to their quest for love. Children wonder why Daddy or Mommy didn't love them enough to keep their home together. Parents in their old age wonder where they went wrong when their children don't want to spend time with them. An estranged spouse wonders why his or her marriage partner could have been seduced by "that man" or "that woman." We cannot hope to find answers for the painful questions of life without first discovering the source of love.

GOD IS LOVE

The Bible doesn't simply say that God *loves* or that He *has* love; it states plainly, "God *is* love" (1 John 4:8, emphasis added). His very essence is divine love, which He desires to infuse into all of His creation. Is it any wonder that the human heart craves love so deeply and on so many levels? We were made by love to walk in relationship with God, who is love. Seeking God, who *is* love, to come into our lives and dwell there is one of the most awesome spiritual realities we can experience. Learning to appreciate God's presence in our lives is the first step in knowing true satisfaction for our deepest desire for love.

A Hebrew verb for *love* is *ahab* and means to have affection for, as for a friend.[1] Our whole being—heart, soul, and strength—is to be engaged in cultivating friendship with God. Only in that divine relationship can we expect to find ultimate satisfaction in life. Love is to be the motivating force for humanity.

The Bible is filled with revelation of the kind of intimacy God desires to have with mankind. The writer of the Proverbs declared, "For the devious are an abomination to the LORD; but He is intimate with the upright" (Prov. 3:32, NASB). In Hebrew the word *intimate* means to sit down together, to counsel and instruct, to establish, to settle, and to share inward secrets.[2] To think of sitting down with God and receiving His counsel, and even hearing His secrets, may seem almost irreverent to some. But for those who are learning to appreciate the Creator and who have felt His divine presence, even as they observe His awesome creation, it is the most deeply satisfying experience they have known.

Our deep craving for intimacy involves the innate need to be fully known, fully loved, and fully accepted. At every stage of life, we encounter different need loves, pleasures of appreciation, and expressions of gift love. The very young have need loves that can be fulfilled by those who are more mature, expressing gift love toward them. And the elderly once again experience some of the need loves of children, which can be fulfilled by young people sharing their love for them. There must be a balance in all of life for expressing the natural loves, which of course must be submitted to God's divine love. As we seek God to anoint our lives with His love, the natural loves will take on godly character and will help us fulfill the destiny for which we were ordained.

PERSONAL REFLECTION

_____

_____

_____

_____

_____

DAY 16

SALVATION OF MANKIND

G OD IS THE creative genius of all that scientists are only recently discovering in astounding detail under high-powered microscopes and through powerful telescopes. When God created mankind, He placed Adam and Eve in a beautiful garden. They were given dominion over all of creation and the task of tending the garden. Their greater purpose was to enjoy communion with God continuously.

Tragically, through mankind's determined disobedience to the laws of creation given by the Creator, we suffered the loss of that intimate relationship. As a result, this alienation from our Creator-God became a tragic reality, not just for that first couple but for all mankind.

God knew before He formed man that He would lose the precious relationship He delighted in and enjoyed with the first couple, Adam and Eve. Scripture clearly states that God's remedy for mankind's disobedience was already in place at the time of creation.

In the Book of Revelation, Christ is called "the Lamb slain from the foundation of the world" (13:8). To enjoy the "family" He wanted, God knew, even before He created mankind, that He would have to sacrifice His only begotten Son. Yet so great was His desire to express His love in a reciprocal manner with mankind that He chose to endure the suffering our redemption would require.

It will perhaps require all of eternity for us to appreciate the profound sacrifice that Christ, the Son of God, became for us at Calvary. The fact of His crucifixion and the unimaginable suffering and agony in the manner of His death is terrible enough. Yet we must consider that this was the Lamb of God, the perfect One, who had never known the terrible curse of sin. Yet He *became* sin for us so that we could be freed from its curse (2 Cor. 5:21). We can only bow our heads and our hearts at the foot of the cross and worship in deep gratitude for the peace of God we enjoy as believers because Christ loved us enough to lay down His life for us.

ETERNAL LIFE

All of Scripture reveals the heart of our eternal Father, who longs to enjoy fellowship with His highest creation, mankind, forever. Simply stated, eternal life is *knowing* God. To know Him involves properly appreciating who He is, who He made you to be, and all that He has given you for life. As we continually yield our lives to Christ, we can enjoy the quality of eternal life now, in this troubled world, which will prepare our hearts to live with God forever. These desirable qualities of eternal life are described in Scripture as peace, joy, righteousness, strength, and rest for our souls. Love, patience, perseverance, and every other named characteristic of God are worked in us as we yield our souls to His redemptive process, seeking Him to anoint our hearts and lives.

There are those who dare not assert that they will live with God forever; they cling to a vague hope that if they are a good person, everything is all right between them and God. That is not the teaching of Scripture. Being born again into relationship with God is a decisive experience, followed by cultivating a new lifestyle of obedience to the Word of God. For believers, life becomes an adventure into truth and a satisfying relationship with the One who made them. It was John who made it supremely clear that we can know that we have eternal life: "These things I have written to you who believe in the name of the Son of God, that you may know that you have eternal life, and that you may continue to believe in the name of the Son of God" (1 John 5:13).

The supreme love of our heavenly Father permeates every facet of redemption. So great is the gift of His salvation of our souls that Scripture declares even angels desire to look into it (1 Pet. 1:12).

PERSONAL REFLECTION

_____

_____

_____

_____

_____

_____

_____

_____

_____

DAY 17

FORGIVENESS

ALTHOUGH IT IS true that we receive forgiveness of our sins through the shed blood of Jesus Christ, forgiveness is not introduced first to New Testament believers. Forgiveness is taught clearly in the Old Testament as well. Ever since Adam and Eve sinned in the Garden of Eden, which blinded them to a relationship with God, God has been offering His forgiveness to those who have sinned against Him.

For some, forgiveness of sin simply seems more than they can hope for. There are people who believe in Christ and His sacrifice on the cross but feel they are "too bad," their sin is too awful, and they don't deserve to be forgiven. The wonder of divine grace is that no one deserves to receive it; it is unmerited favor. Grace is a divine gift given by a loving God to a sinful world. The good news of the gospel is that "while we were still sinners, Christ died for us" (Rom. 5:8). Such is the unfathomable love of God. It is no wonder that when we experience salvation, we can only bow in worship before Him.

Some have not entered into the spiritual freedom that forgiveness brings because they cannot forgive themselves. R. T. Kendall, the pastor of Westminster Chapel in London for twenty-five years, discussed this in a powerful book he wrote called *Total Forgiveness*.

Forgiveness is worthless to us emotionally if we can't forgive ourselves....It certainly isn't *total* forgiveness unless we forgive ourselves as well as others. God knows this. This is why He wants us to forgive ourselves as well as to accept His promise that our past is under the blood of Christ....He wants to make it easy for us to forgive ourselves.[1]

Others describe this concept as really and truly believing our own sins are totally forgiven, that between God and our souls everything is cleared away. Each time we pray, we can ask the Father to forgive us for our sin. And we must expect that He will be true to His Word and do it. If you have difficulty forgiving yourself or others, I encourage you to begin to thank God in faith for the promise of His Word. As you do, the power of the Holy Spirit will be manifest in your life to make forgiveness a reality to your heart, cleansing you and filling you with His peace and joy.

Another reason that people sometimes do not enjoy the spiritual freedom of total forgiveness is that they have not forgiven others who have hurt them. Do you remember the phrase in the model prayer, "Forgive us our debts, as we forgive our debtors"? (See Matthew 6:9–13.) To enjoy spiritual freedom, you must choose to forgive those you consider your "debtors." As R. T. Kendall explains, people who offend, hurt, and wound you deeply must receive your forgiveness for you to be free.

When everything in you wants to hold a grudge, point a finger and remember the pain, God wants you to lay it all aside. You can avoid spiritual quicksand and experience the incredible freedom found in total forgiveness.[2]

After Jesus taught the disciples to pray the model prayer, He continued to talk to them about their need to forgive others.

> For if you forgive men their trespasses, your heavenly Father will also forgive you. But if you do not forgive men their trespasses, neither will your Father forgive your trespasses.
>
> —MATTHEW 6:14–15

Some may say they have tried to forgive but cannot rid themselves of the bad feelings and negative thoughts they have toward a person. Forgiveness, like any other godly act, must be done by the grace of God through faith. Forgiveness is a choice, not a feeling. After the right choice is made, feelings will begin to change. As believers, we can be sure that God will not ask us to do something that cannot be done. He is a gracious Father who provides us with all we need to become Christlike.

As we accept the truth of God's Word, which promises "all things work together for good" (Rom. 8:28), it will be easier to release others from our resentment, grudges, and bitterness. These negative emotional responses will do much more harm to ourselves than to anyone else. Unforgiveness will destroy you, your relationship with the Lord, and your relationship with those around you.

The Scriptures demonstrate that it is possible to face bitter experiences of life without becoming bitter, negative people. The grace of God will keep you in perfect peace as your mind is continually meditating on His love. As you choose to forgive, you will enjoy the complete forgiveness of the Father. And He will manifest His divine power in your soul to cleanse your heart from all negative feelings and thoughts toward others.

PERSONAL REFLECTION

_____

_____

_____

_____

_____

_____

_____

_____

_____

_____

_____

_____

_____

_____

_____

_____

_____

_____

Day 18

Grace

THE DIVINE GRACE of God, which can be translated as "favor," was first revealed in the Old Testament to the people of God. For example, Scripture declares, "Noah found grace in the eyes of the LORD" (Gen. 6:8). When the patriarch Abraham was visited by the Lord, he said, "My Lord, if I have now found favor [grace] in Your sight, do not pass on by Your servant" (Gen. 18:3). The Hebrew word for *grace* or *favor* used in these and other passages comes from the word *chanan* (khaw-nan`), which gives a wonderful word picture of the grace and favor of God. It literally means "to bend or stoop in kindness to an inferior; to favor, bestow [good upon]."[1]

As created beings, we are inferior to the Creator who made us. Yet in His great kindness, He stoops down to give us His favor, to bestow His divine grace and kindness upon us. The goodness of God is beyond anything we can ever imagine. Nothing compares to His love, His peace, His prosperity—the total well-being of body, mind, and spirit that He wants His children to experience.

Unfortunately our human minds often cannot conceive of God without inadvertently "pulling Him down" to our size, making Him one of us. When we consider the grace of God, we must understand it is unlike any *human* characteristic we have observed or experienced.

Meditating on the divine favor of God can fill our hearts

56

with wonder and gratitude for His love for us. In the New Testament the Greek word *charis* is translated "grace." It means "favor, joy, pleasure, and the divine influence upon the heart and its reflection in the life." A life that is filled with the grace of God will reflect all of these wonderful qualities of life.

Jesus declared, "Therefore if the Son makes you free, you shall be free indeed" (John 8:36). "Free indeed" is a wonderful description of a life filled with the grace and favor of God. For believers, remembering our rescue from slavery to sin should fill us with continual gratitude.

As finite human beings, we cannot expect to fully grasp the profound grace that caused Christ to come to earth as a man and lay down His life for us. Yet we can revel in the wonder of His coming and be filled with gratitude for the saving grace He has made available to us.

Not only does the grace of God save us from sin; it also keeps us in the love of God, protecting us from the destructive forces that come into our lives through daily challenges. The apostle Peter understood that we are "kept by the power of God through faith" (1 Pet. 1:5). And the apostle Paul declared, "By the grace of God I am what I am" (1 Cor. 15:10). He wrote to Titus of the keeping power of that grace: "For the grace of God that brings salvation has appeared to all men…that He might redeem us from every lawless deed and purify for Himself His own special people, zealous for good works" (Titus 2:11, 14). Whatever the temptations or trials we face in life, the Word of God promises that God's grace is sufficient to help us conquer them. (See 2 Corinthians 12:9.)

THRONE OF GOD

Scripture teaches that there is a place to receive the grace of God—the throne of God. While we are not accustomed, as Americans, to relating to royalty, in biblical times people were quite aware of the awesome presence of kings who ruled with absolute power from their thrones. The reigning monarch had authority to do what he would with his subjects, which often caused them to live in fear.

Thankfully we don't have a King who threatens us with possible death when we come into His presence. On the contrary, Jesus Christ, who is called the King of kings, is sitting at the right hand of the throne of God, making intercession for us (Rom. 8:34). He welcomes us into His presence, telling us to cast all of our care on Him because He cares for us. (See 1 Peter 5:7.) And He assures us that as we come to His throne of grace, we will find help in our time of need (Heb. 4:16).

As you meditate on the grace of God, dear reader, I encourage you to approach His throne of grace boldly to receive His divine favor for whatever your need is this day. There you will find the answer to the longing of your heart. And the peace that only God can give will bless your life—spirit, soul, and body.

PERSONAL REFLECTION

_____

_____

_____

_____

Day 19

Guarding Our Faith

I N ITS ESSENCE faith is simply crediting or accepting God's testimony. According to Scripture, if we do not believe the witness of God, we make Him a liar (1 John 5:9–10). And if we believe God's testimony, essentially it means that we believe and trust in "the Son of God; for He, and salvation in Him alone, form the grand subject of God's testimony. The Holy Spirit alone enables any man to accept God's testimony and accept Jesus Christ as his divine Savior" (1 John 5:11–13). Faith is receiving "God's gratuitous gift of eternal life in Christ."[1]

Enemies of the Faith

The apostle Paul's counsel to the young man, Timothy, was to "fight the good fight of faith, lay hold on eternal life, to which you were also called" (1 Tim. 6:12). He was acknowledging the fact that there are enemies to our faith that would love to defeat us in life. Let's look quickly at three key enemies to our faith.

1. Unbelief

Jesus Himself came to His own country and, according to Scripture, "could do no mighty work there" (Mark 6:5). The people knew Jesus as the young carpenter, the son of Mary, and were offended at Him. And Scripture says that Jesus marveled at their unbelief (Mark 6:6). The divine Son of God left his friends and neighbors in unbelief and would not perform miracles among them. It is dangerous to dishonor the Son of God through unbelief!

The solution to our unbelief is to fill our hearts and minds with the Word of God, which is the source of faith (Rom. 10:17). While saving faith is initially a gift of God to those who seek it, believers must continually seek to know Him through His Word and through communion in prayer so that their faith will grow. Only in that way can we displace unbelief more and more in our lives.

As our appreciation for God increases, we will find our faith increased to help us win the battle against unbelief. The importance of strengthening our faith cannot be overemphasized, for without it we cannot please God (Heb. 11:6).

2. Common sense

Perhaps an even more subtle enemy to faith is what we call "plain common sense." We use this phrase to refer to a situation where you do not ignore the obvious realities staring you in the face. Considering natural circumstances and making decisions accordingly seems to be the practical way to live life. That may be true for the natural person, but it does not work in the realm of spiritual realities.

When we have spiritual sight, there is a spiritual "common sense" that does not forget God's promise, God's Word, and God's work. Remember the biblical definition of faith: "Now faith is the substance of things hoped for, the evidence of things not seen" (Heb. 11:1). Faith has spiritual eyes to see what has not yet been manifested in our natural circumstances as the will of God for our lives. With faith we choose to believe what God promises to do even before He does it.

3. The devil

There is another enemy to our faith that will never give up trying to defeat us—the devil. Scripture clearly teaches that the devil has come to kill, steal, and destroy. (See John 10:10.) Peter describes him as a "roaring lion, seeking whom he may devour" (1 Pet. 5:8). Yet the Word of God also teaches us that Satan was defeated at Calvary and that we can walk in victory over his attacks: "Submit to God. Resist the devil and he will flee from you" (James 4:7).

One of the most powerful prayers the apostle Paul prayed was for believers to grow in their faith in order to experience all God has for them (Eph. 3:14–19). I encourage you to read this prayer and to meditate on the promises it offers the believer. As believers prayerfully seek to know Christ dwelling in their hearts through *faith*, they can come to know the love of Christ in a most profound way. And we can be filled with all the fullness of God. Growing in faith offers us the supernatural benefits of being strengthened by the Holy Spirit, experiencing the riches of His glory, and becoming rooted and grounded in the divine love of God. In this way we will also learn to walk in unity with our brothers and sisters within the body of Christ.

PERSONAL REFLECTION

_____

_____

_____

_____

_____

DAY 20

SURRENDER TO GOD

THE DEFINITION OF *surrender* is "to yield to the power, control, or possession of another...to give up completely or agree to forgo in favor of another."[1] We are called to surrender our lives to God, accepting Christ as our Savior. (See Mark 8:34.) Without the working of the Holy Spirit in our lives, that surrender would not be possible. Choosing to enter into relationship with God, by the power of the Holy Spirit, we receive new desires to be wholly united with and surrendered to our benevolent Creator.

When we offer our lives to God through the redeeming work of Christ, we discover the sheer joy of *relinquishment*. As we focus our attentions on His majesty and bring all our thoughts and desires into alignment with His divine will for our lives, we become intoxicated with the lovely fragrance of the peace of relinquishment. Nothing makes our prayers as sweet as coming before the Lord, surrendering to His will alone, and asking for His help to get through a painful trial.

Suffering life's trials often brings us to a greater surrender to our Lord. When we as believers enter into intimate communion with God, making Him the essence of our lives, when we have lost *everything* that was of value to us—in that place of total surrender, we experience the unutterable sweetness of relinquishment. Then we realize that the things of the world were not important to our fulfillment. Our greatest joy is to honor God by surrendering to our Creator-Redeemer.

Following Christ wholeheartedly will result in a life filled with purpose, meaning, love, and divine blessing. Conversely, choosing to follow our own desires and "have it our way" will result in the misery that comes from living a selfish, self-centered life, which ultimately attacks itself, ending in self-destruction.

God will enable you to surrender your life more and more to Him as you sincerely seek Him. It is a process as you build your relationship with God.[2] As a believer, you have the life of Christ, who lived a life of complete surrender to the Father, dwelling in you. He is living in your heart through the power of the Holy Spirit, and He will draw you to surrender to the Father, energizing you with holy desires for God. God Himself helps you to put your trust in Him and relinquish your life to His divine destiny for you.

If you determine not to trust in your own strength, but to fix your sights on God's majesty, you will enjoy a heart that is relinquished to God, trusting Him, and depending on Him for all He has promised to give to those who trust Him.

True Joy and Rest

Joy is a wonderful characteristic of the surrendered life. Indeed, it is difficult to imagine a joy-filled life without absolute surrender to God. Jesus clearly teaches the prerequisites for experiencing His joy. It is a result of cultivating relationship with Him (John 15:11). That request is filled with promise of leading us into a life filled with well-being, success, delight, and a continual state of happiness. He is asking believers to live in complete surrender to God as He lived in total surrender to His Father.

Our Redeemer is the only source of true joy. True joy depends on total abandonment to God and His sovereignty.

Christ describes our relationship as joy being made full. We have a new spirit of joy, love, forgiveness, peace, and generosity. We have new imaginations that transform us internally and change the quality of our relationships with others. The fruit of the Spirit (Gal. 5:22–23) is God at work in us, producing the supernatural attributes of Christ in our lives. We cannot develop these qualities fully by ourselves but only through our union with Christ. Our joy is having joy in Him.[3]

Rest is another wonderful result of living a completely surrendered life to God. The promise of profound rest of soul is found only in abandoning our lives to Jesus, choosing to receive the promises of His redemption. He will teach us how to think and how to respond, and He will remove fear and other negative emotions from our minds and hearts.

As we learn to rest in His redemption, we will experience His joy, and we will leave worldly pursuits behind. As we focus on His sweet will for our lives, we will realize that what we own in life is not important. Taking on the mind-set of Jesus, surrendering to His will, transforms our priorities. We take on Jesus Himself as our portion; we see life differently.[4]

PERSONAL REFLECTION

_____

_____

_____

_____

_____

Day 21

Peace

There are so many different reasons for worry. Too often we consider worry a legitimate emotional response to life. Yet if we continually give in to anxiety and worry as part of our emotional "lifestyle," we can never know the wonderful peace God came to give us. But if we seek God, He will *multiply* His peace to us.

Of course there can be no true peace without first being reconciled to relationship with God. Scripture clearly teaches that we can only find true peace for our spirit, soul, and body in personal relationship with God. According to Scripture, it is the will of God that you live in serenity of mind and heart—the harmony and tranquility that allows your body to function at optimum health. Peace is one of the greatest blessings of salvation. And peace is perhaps one of the most longed-for states of mind for millions of people who are looking for it in all the wrong places.

It is a deception to think that financial security, relational happiness, fame, or the fulfillment of any other desire of the heart can, in itself, produce peace. This painful deception has caused many to waste their lives seeking these things in vain in their search for the peace that only God can give.

Peace is not a passive state of mind in which we sit back and allow life to go by. Peace is a positive perspective of life that allows us to be at our best in the situations where Christ has placed us to accomplish His work.

Think about the places God has placed you—your neighborhood, church, school, or workplace. Now think about the growing need in our society for the true peace of God. The mass shootings, terrorist attacks, and natural disasters our country has experienced over the last few decades have been devastating events, affecting families, communities, and entire regions with grief and loss. These troubled times demand a renewed effort to seek peace from a source other than natural circumstances.

The secret to finding peace in the midst of great trouble and sorrow is to call on God. Though it may seem difficult to be thankful in the midst of great loss, as believers, we can express our gratitude for the ability to look up to God and expect Him to help us. As we cultivate a thankful heart, we will be engulfed in the Lord's presence, which will bring His peace and comfort to our aching hearts. The simple act of thanksgiving brings us into the presence of God, who will give us hope and provision for our future.

The apostle Paul declared that the peace of God surpasses all understanding. (See Philippians 4:7.) Even when we cannot make sense of life's circumstances, we can walk in the peace of God by faith, knowing that He loves us and will look out for our welfare. Jesus told His disciples that He was giving them His peace, which would remain even in face of the troubled world in which they lived (John 16:33).

We need this transcending power of the peace of God in our troubled world today. As we accept this promise by faith, we learn to appropriate the peace of God to our personal circumstances. There is no situation so terrible that God's peace cannot permeate it.

CHRIST IS OUR PEACE

At Christ's birth the angelic hosts proclaimed to the shepherds: "Glory to God in the highest, and on earth peace, goodwill toward men!" (Luke 2:14). The coming of the Messiah offered peace to the whole world and harmony between the peoples of the earth. This wonderful, divine gift of peace to the world was prophesied hundreds of years earlier by the Old Testament prophets (Isa. 9:6).

We understand from Scripture that a day is coming when all wars will cease (Isa. 2:4). Yet even Jesus prophesied that the world would be filled with wars and rumors of wars before His second coming. (See Matthew 24.) This is why He has given believers His peace that passes understanding to help us cope in this troubled world.

Scripture teaches that we must *pursue* peace if we are to enjoy its wonderful benefits (Heb. 12:14; 1 Pet. 3:10–11). Our peace depends on entering into God's method of fulfilling His purposes in our lives so we can glorify Him. As we become one with His intention, we can pursue the things the Lord wants us to do. Surely in our troubled world today this divine gift of peace is a treasure worth pursuing.

PERSONAL REFLECTION

_____

_____

_____

_____

Day 22

A Garden of Prayer

S CRIPTURE DESCRIBES THE people of God as a spiritual garden, filled with thanksgiving, joy, and gladness (Isa. 51:3). We can consider our hearts as gardens in which lovely flowers grow. If we ask God to plant the flowers of truth, peace, and love in our hearts—our spiritual gardens—our lives will reflect the beauty and fragrance of these godly qualities.

As we cultivate the soil of our hearts, asking God to manifest His divine characteristics to flourish there, we prepare a beautiful garden for the Lord to come and commune with us, and we with Him. Filled with appreciation for our Creator, our lives yield the fragrance of thanksgiving, praise, and surrender to His will. Let's take a closer look at five aspects of prayer as we seek to cultivate a garden of prayer in our hearts.

1. **Worship.** True worship is the highest expression of appreciation. Every expression of prayer, whether it is personal communion, petition with thanksgiving, or unselfish intercession, has its basis in worship. Worship is a much more profound relationship than we experience in any earthly relationship. When we acknowledge our Creator, we begin to see His power and glory and grace. We behold His countenance, and we are overwhelmed by His majesty. Our only response is to fall at His feet and worship.[1]

2. **Praise.** Scripture is filled with commands for the people of God to praise Him, such as in Psalm 100:1–5. When I express gratitude and praise, I feel closer to God than I do at other times. I just thank Him, knowing my lack and His greatness. He is from the beginning of time and all through eternity, and yet He is at the center of my "little" life. I have experienced moments in which I have become engaged in a "thanksgiving frenzy." At those times I am truly able to let all earthly concerns go. In this wonderful place of abandonment to God, I can gauge how close I am to Him as I leave behind all other concerns. This attitude of praise is a mental attitude of continual thanks to God that permeates our thoughts and lives. It engulfs our relationship with God, our relationships with others, and our relationship with our vocation.[2]

3. **Petition.** Choosing to believe God's wonderful promises, we can learn to come to Him as our loving Father, Savior, and friend. With thanksgiving for all He is and what He has already done for us, we can present our requests or petitions to Him. As we seek to rest in His redemption, we cease from worrying and fretting, knowing that our loving God will respond to our requests and intervene in our lives with His good will.

4. **Communion.** Although the verb *commune* is used only a few times in Scripture, it is of great significance when describing God's relationship to His people. When God gave Moses the plan to build the ark of the covenant, He promised to commune with

him there (Exod. 25:22). It is difficult to comprehend that the infinite, almighty God—the Creator of the universe—desires to come into our lives in a tangible way and commune with us. Yet that reality has been experienced by many believers who dare to take God at His Word. Satisfaction comes through daily communion with God. He wants an intimate relationship of love with us. And Christ is the key to that intimacy. Our relationship with Christ is to be one of surrender, filled with desire to have intimate fellowship with Him until we are engulfed in and intertwined with His presence. Then we enter into the fullness of God![3]

5. **Intercession.** We are called to intercede for others—to pray fervently for one another. It is not always easy to be a loving intercessor. There are times when others are difficult to deal with. They may be filled with anger, worry, cynicism, or other negative attitudes, but we need to be continuously filled with the Holy Spirit, praying even for those who "use" us, hate us, and act against us.[4] As we become more and more filled with the love of God, we will feel His love for others who are hurting. In that way we learn to become intercessors for them rather than accusers.

Ask God to give you a concern for another person and help you to *intercede* for the person's needs. And take time to quietly *commune* with God, expecting to hear His response to your desire and to feel Him near. Bow before Him in *praise* and *worship* for who He is. Make your *petitions* known to Him, for He delights in giving good gifts to His children.

PERSONAL REFLECTION

_____

_____

_____

_____

_____

_____

_____

_____

_____

_____

_____

_____

_____

_____

_____

_____

_____

Day 23

Divine Testing

S OMETIMES WE ARE faced with trials of serious health issues, financial crises, devastating relational problems, or other troubles. And we observe friends and family who are going through difficult experiences as well. These challenges present themselves at every stage of life. During these painful times, which the Bible refers to as *trials* or *tests*, it is most important for us to engage in the grace of appreciation, adoration, and awe for our Creator.

Trials—whether defined by illness, financial problems, relationship problems, great emotional loss, or other painful situations—require us to rely more on God and not on worldly sources for strength and comfort. When I am tempted to be discouraged in the face of a trial, I love to read the promise of God found in Romans 8:28:

> And we know that all things work together for good to those who love God, to those who are the called according to His purpose.

Intimacy With God

If there is anything that can comfort the human heart in a time of difficulty and trial, it is enjoying the *intimacy* of a loving relationship with God. As you seek to know God personally, you will discover that you can always live in God's presence.

This divine perspective changes the dynamic of every trial you must face in life. God truly becomes a refuge for believers in our times of trouble.

It is a sad reality that it often takes a severe trial to draw us to God. Often we have to suffer the pangs of personal trials before we can become open and transparent before God, laying hold of the restoring "glue" of His grace, forgiveness, compassion, and comfort. In our pain we look up and realize that God is waiting for us to call on Him for help. When we do, we experience a divine melding of our souls with God, through the cross and Christ's forgiveness, which fills us with His divine comfort. As believers, that divine love and grace permeate our beings and then flow out to bless others we encounter.

Paradoxically the pain that believers suffer through trials allows the wonderful grace and comfort of God to be revealed to us and through us in deeper ways. It is simply a fact of human nature that when we feel strong and have no need of help beyond ourselves, we do not seek the Lord. We usually have to be brought down by the pain of trials to become as children, crying out to God for help and comfort. In our pain we are willing to forsake our busyness and activities that keep us from seeking God. We lay aside our pride and arrogance that can be associated with traditional religion. It is in our painful trials that we best learn to lean on God in total dependence.

In that place of humble abandonment to the will of God, we discover the wonderful secrets of His tender care. Our attitude in these difficult times is to be one of rejoicing, putting our faith in the divine power of our God that will keep us from harm.

According to Scripture, these trials of our faith are "more precious than gold" (1 Pet. 1:6–7), giving opportunity for us to humble ourselves before God. What a wonderful truth we can embrace, that we can cast all our care upon God because He cares for us. Humility is required for us to give our troubles to God and ask for His help. Otherwise, we will strive to solve our problems in our own strength.

While Scripture does not promise immunity from trouble for the believer in Christ, it does show us how our gratitude and appreciation for our Creator can give us a wonderful life perspective in the face of trials. As we turn to God in our trials, they will work in us an "eternal weight of glory." The glory of God is His divine presence, which He wants our lives to reflect. On another occasion, Paul declared that it is "Christ in you, the hope of glory" (Col. 1:27). Growing in our relationship with God through trials will reveal the presence and glory of God to us and through us.

Bowing before God in adoration and worship, casting our care on Him, and seeking His divine help will cause us to grow in the grace of humility. Our minds will be transformed to become Christlike as we trust Him in the trials of our lives. And in that transformation we will discover divine destiny— the purpose for which we were born. Then our gratitude for God's love shown to us deepens further still.

PERSONAL REFLECTION

_____

_____

_____

_____

_____

Day 24
Divine Destiny

Gᴏᴅ'ꜱ ᴘʟᴀɴ ꜰᴏʀ your life, your divine destiny, is what I call your "Christian manifesto." As you surrender your life to the blessed Holy Spirit, He will teach you to develop the character and the abilities you need to fulfill the divine purpose for which you were born. What you *do* can never define who you *are*. As believers, we become sons and daughters of God and find our significance and fulfillment in relationship with our Creator alone. He who made us unique individuals is also delighting in our fulfillment of personal destiny.

Part of glorifying God and enjoying Him forever involves the satisfaction of what you do every day in the workplace. There you learn to appreciate your anointed purpose for life, accepting it as a blessed gift from God. It is in the daily duties of chosen employment or vocation where a sense of significance, valuable relationships, and the satisfaction of personal challenges can be realized.

For some, that workplace may be the home where you nurture and care for your family. For others, your workplace may be the farm, a factory, a corporate business, a store, a school, a hospital, an emergency response team, an athletics facility, the military, a research laboratory—or a myriad of other jobs and professions needed within our society.

The important thing to consider in choosing your workplace is that you are not simply looking for a job. If you want to know true fulfillment in life, you must first seek personal relationship with God. In cultivating that relationship, you will discover His hand guiding you regarding your place of employment, relationships, and every other issue of life.

Sometimes your Christian manifesto means simply being a servant, living without acclaim, and walking in satisfying relationship with God as you complete your daily tasks. It is asking God to live out His life in you, whatever the nature of your vocation, profession, or work.

It is in cultivating relationship with your Creator that you will find the true meaning of life, not in the fortunes that you amass. He will reveal your unique purpose for life, which will guarantee personal fulfillment as a unique servant of God.

Surrendering your agenda and desires to God requires a willingness to serve others. If you desire the beauty of character of your Master and Savior, Jesus Christ, you will have to have His attitude toward others. Jesus, the Master, took a towel and a basin and washed His disciples' feet. We must cultivate that same humble attitude of servanthood in our lives, surrendering ourselves to become people who delight in caring for the most mundane needs of others. Godly humility grows in our hearts as we continue to develop a life perspective of gratitude for our Creator.

Fulfilling your Christian manifesto in the workplace means learning to appreciate your employers, coworkers, clients, and customers. You can even appreciate the difficulties of a seventy-hour workweek or other "negatives" you encounter as you determine to serve the Lord in love. The attitude of a servant is never hostile or lazy; it is conciliatory and selfless, intent on fulfilling the task at hand to the best of one's ability. You must determine that your attitudes and actions toward others are ethical and, above all, kind.

It is also important to look in the mirror and encourage yourself. You don't have to live in fear, guilt, or remorse over past failures; you simply need to ask God for forgiveness. As you receive His cleansing through the blood of Christ, you will learn how to draw near to Him. You will know the fulfillment of living in dependence on Him.

As you discover your Christian manifesto, you will learn to trust God for your financial provisions. Of course it is helpful to develop your skills and abilities to the highest level possible in the workplace, but there will always be factors beyond your control that affect your ability to earn a living. The economy, your health, and even politics in the workplace can sometimes hinder your success. However, as you learn to walk in dependence upon God, you will discover that He is your Jehovah Jireh—the Lord your Provider.

It is never too late, even if you have spent a lifetime being unhappy in your work, to begin seeking God. As you surrender your life to God, either He will open doors to another kind of employment, or He will empower you to change your attitude and become content and fulfilled where you are.

True fulfillment, as we have discussed, comes from knowing God. Cultivating that divine relationship changes your perspective of all of life. Ultimately your Christian manifesto can be fulfilled only as far as you surrender to become conformed to the image of our Lord Jesus Christ.

PERSONAL REFLECTION

_____

_____

_____

Day 25
Divine Rest

I N THE BIBLICAL account of the beginning, or genesis, of life as we know it, God established a law and a pattern of rest for His creation. After He finished His work of creation, the Genesis account declares: "And on the seventh day God ended His work which He had done, and He rested on the seventh day from all His work which He had done" (Gen. 2:2). Was He fatigued? Did He need to sleep? No. It would be unthinkable for an omnipotent God to become weary. Yet God built into all of creation an inherent need for rest—that is, for complete cessation from activity to allow for a time of "re-creation."

The Hebrew word *shabath* is where we get the word *Sabbath*, meaning "to repose, desist from exertion, cease, and celebrate."[1] And in the Law of Moses, the fourth commandment declares, "Remember the Sabbath day, to keep it holy" (Exod. 20:8).

If we embrace the fact that God has blessed the Sabbath day and choose to abide by that "rest principle," we can be the beneficiaries of the blessing God intended the Sabbath to be for all creation. God's law regarding the Sabbath rest was not meant to be a burden to us but a joy; it was given by a loving Creator, who understands the needs of His creation. He established a Sabbath rest to ensure our freedom from sickness and other ills.

Our bodies, our psyches, and our spirits must have proper times of rest so that we don't "burn out." Resting re-creates strength in life; it is necessary to every area of our health. In every area of life, we must consider the God-given need for rest of body, mind, and spirit.

To seek divine rest is a determined choice Christians have to make as we face the overwhelming conflicts of daily life. We must throw all of our care upon Him because He cares for us (1 Pet. 5:7). Choosing to rely on Christ alone in all of life's situations will teach us how to always rely on Him, especially in difficult situations with which we cannot cope. It is exhilarating to see the hand of God move into a situation and change it in ways we could never have done.

The most important aspect of rest is *inner* rest. More than simply an outward cessation from activity, the rest we need is spiritual. As we wait on God and fill our minds with His Word, we are enabled to trust His love with even the most devastating situations we face.

Whereas the need for physical rest and freedom from the tensions of life in order to enjoy true rest for our physical bodies has long been established, on a deeper level inner rest is the state of mind in which we can be truly happy in Christ. Emotional and spiritual contentment depend on being at peace with God and with ourselves to such an extent that we need nothing else to stimulate our happiness. We cease to look for satisfaction in all the wrong places and discover complete fulfillment in our relationship with our Creator.

Balance is required to experience rest for our souls. Surrender to our divine destiny in vocation and work will help to affect this balance. Taking time for rest and recreation will also create balance. Perhaps most important, however, is that we learn to rest in God—in His redemption. As we seek mental and emotional satisfaction through study of the Word of God, prayer, and communion with Him, we will discover

His wonderful provision for all our needs. And we will not "suffer" a sense of lack, which seeks to be satisfied with apparent happiness from lesser sources. Instead, we will deepen our sense of gratitude for the love of our God and the happiness He brings into our lives.

I wish everyone could enjoy this divine promise for perfect balance and well-being. This profound, inner rest from mental, emotional, and relational conflicts promised in Scripture sounds almost too good to be true. But for one who dares to seek God, to wait on Him, and to fill his or her mind with the truth of God's Word, the divine rest of God will increasingly rule in every dimension of life. Pursuing a relationship with God will create a divine balance for all of life. And that balance will bring profound rest to your life.

PERSONAL REFLECTION

_____

_____

_____

_____

_____

_____

_____

_____

_____

Day 26

Divine Comfort

E MOTIONAL LOSS, BROKEN hearts, mental anguish—all of these are part of the human experience; no one is exempt. After suffering the painful loss of a loved one, we often hear the timeworn cliché "Time heals all wounds." Unfortunately the experience of many is that even if the passage of time dulls the ache, they never really "get over" their loss; they just learn to manage their pain. Some look for "escapes" with alcohol or tranquilizers, activities, or other relationships. Sadly they never appreciate the wonderful promise and power of divine comfort offered to us in Scripture and realized by many believers who testify of its healing power.

By definition, *comfort* is "consolation in time of trouble or worry; solace; a feeling of relief or encouragement; contented well-being; a satisfying or enjoyable experience."[1] *Solace*, a synonym for *comfort*, means "alleviation of grief or anxiety; a source of relief or consolation."[2] As we learn to receive the tangible comfort of God offered in Scripture, our hearts will be filled with joy and contentment, even in the face of life's painful realities and losses.

OUR SHEPHERD

The twenty-third psalm, one of the most beloved of all the psalms, paints a beautiful picture of our Lord as a Shepherd, full of comfort and all that is needed to satisfy His sheep.

Countless people of every nation on earth have found this
endearing analogy of our Lord to be a healing balm, a real
comfort, in their time of sorrow and pain. I am convinced that
if you take a moment to declare reverently, "The Lord is *my*
Shepherd," you will experience the comfort of God.

Jesus referred to Himself as the Good Shepherd (John 10:14),
and He referred to His followers as sheep. And He promised
that He will provide all that His followers need to experience
freedom from the anxieties of life that keep us from "lying
down in green pastures." In a personal relationship with Christ,
we have everything we need for true satisfaction. He continually offers the blessings of His *provision, protection, peace, joy,*
and, most of all, His divine *presence* to guide and comfort those
who love Him. Here are just a few of those precious promises
that offer profound comfort for all who will receive it:

- **Presence.** "Jesus answered and said to him,
  'If anyone loves Me, he will keep My word;
  and My Father will love him, and We will
  come to him and make Our home with him'"
  (John 14:23).

- **Provision.** "Therefore do not worry, saying,
  'What shall we eat?' or 'What shall we
  drink?'...For your heavenly Father knows
  that you need all these things. But seek first
  the kingdom of God and His righteousness,
  and all these things shall be added to you"
  (Matt. 6:31–33).

- **Protection.** "Holy Father, keep through
  Your name those whom You have given Me,

that they may be one as We are....I do not
pray for these alone, but also for those who
will believe in Me through their word" (John
17:11, 20).

- **Peace.** "Peace I leave with you, My peace I
  give to you; not as the world gives do I give to
  you. Let not your heart be troubled, neither
  let it be afraid" (John 14:27).

- **Joy.** "These things I have spoken to you, that
  My joy may remain in you, and that your joy
  may be full" (John 15:11).

Jesus understood that we would have problems in this life,
that we would suffer grief and loss. He told His disciples:
"These things I have spoken to you, that in Me you may have
peace. In the world you will have tribulation; but be of good
cheer, I have overcome the world" (John 16:33).

It is awesome to think that the Holy Spirit, God Himself, is
given to us that we might receive the divine comfort we so desperately need in life's most painful circumstances. God's divine
power to give relief from grief and anxiety offers true healing
that time alone cannot give. As we receive Christ as Savior
and trust the Holy Spirit to do His precious work in our lives,
God's presence in our lives heals our minds and hearts and
gives us supernatural peace and joy. This is what the apostle
Paul referred to when he declared: "For the kingdom of God is
not eating and drinking, but righteousness and peace and joy in
the Holy Spirit" (Rom. 14:17). As we continue to discover the
reality of these divine promises, our hearts will overflow with
deep gratitude for our Creator.

PERSONAL REFLECTION

_____

_____

_____

_____

_____

_____

_____

_____

_____

_____

_____

_____

_____

_____

_____

_____

_____

_____

Day 27

MARGIN

In Dr. Richard Swenson's book *Margin: Restoring Emotional, Physical, Financial, and Time Reserves to Overloaded Lives*, he uses the following simple equation to help us define the term *margin*:

DEFINING MARGIN

Power (P) minus Load (L) equals Margin (M); $P - L = M$.

> *Power* is made up of factors, such as skills, time, emotional and physical strength, faith, finances, social supports, and education.
>
> *Load* is made up of such factors as work, problems, obligations and commitments, expectations (internal and external), debt, deadlines, and interpersonal conflicts.[1]

Each person's power to function is different, and it changes during different stages of life, as does the load we carry. What does *not* change is this basic principle relating to margin: "When our load is greater than our power, we enter into negative margin status…we are overloaded." According to Swenson, negative margin for an extended period of time is another name for *burnout*.[2]

Emotional margin

We must be emotionally resilient to "confront our problems with a sense of hope and power." We need to learn which influences drain our emotional batteries and which ones recharge them. For example, when we are sad or angry, frustrated or depressed, our emotional reserves are being spent at a rapid rate. Conversely, if we receive encouragement from significant others or enjoy the satisfaction of completing meaningful activities, our emotional reserves are being replenished.[3]

Among the solutions for restoring margin to emotional energy reserves are establishing the social support of family, friends, community, and church; reconciling relationships; and volunteering to help others. Of course enjoying rest and relaxation, learning to laugh, and allowing ourselves to cry are also extremely helpful. Expressing appreciation, giving thanks, and, above all, giving love are also powerful ways to replenish emotional margin.

Time margin

Accepting personal responsibility for the twenty-four hours a day God gives us is the first step in restoring margin in the area of time. According to family researcher Dolores Curran, four of the top ten family stressors have to do with lack of time: insufficient couple time, insufficient *me* time, insufficient family playtime, and overscheduled family calendars.[4] Dr. James Dobson says, "Crowded lives produce fatigue—and fatigue produces irritability—and irritability produces indifference—and indifference can be interpreted by the child as a lack of genuine affection and personal esteem."[5] Everyone needs personal time, family time, sharing time, and God time.

Some practical suggestions for resolving the problem include: learn to say no, turn off the television, prune back your activity calendar, practice simplicity and contentment, create buffer zones, and plan for free time.[6]

Financial margin

The average credit card debt for the American family stands at more than $8,000.[7] As a culture we have become enamored with "plastic." We consider only whether we can afford the monthly payment, not what the debt will actually cost us after calculating the exorbitant interest rates. We think that to have a financial margin, we simply need to earn more money. The fact is that money *is not* margin. According to Dr. Swenson, establishing a financial margin involves breaking the power money holds on us and learning to use it instead of being used by it.[8] We must walk in appreciation for our Creator's many gifts to us and allow our financial situation to come under His lordship. Laws of biblical finance are clearly taught in Scripture, promising blessing and security to all who will obey them.

A balanced response is the key to recovering healthy margins. Whether you are addressing psychological injuries, emotional hurts, spiritual maladies, or financial woes, finding a balance of priorities is the only way to succeed. Waiting on the Lord, meditating on Scripture, and giving ourselves to prayer will bring to us the supernatural wisdom we need to pursue balance in the exacting challenges of life. We must give God His rightful place at the center of all we are and all we do. As we continue to grow in our appreciation for the Creator's love for us, He teaches us how to live life successfully by maintaining a healthy margin.

PERSONAL REFLECTION

_____

_____

_____

_____

Day 28

Healing

O̲U̲R̲ H̲E̲A̲L̲T̲H̲—O̲U̲R̲ P̲H̲Y̲S̲I̲C̲A̲L̲, mental, and spiritual well-being—is directly related to our relationship with the Creator. If we seek God to receive His anointing on our lives, to live in relationship with Him, and to rest in His redemption, we will enjoy the health He has ordained for us to experience. Our relationship with Christ will fill us with His love and motivate us to care for the gift of life He has given us on every level. Let's look at five levels of healing.

1. Natural healing

Your body was created with an intricate design for health that requires balance. It is so efficient that even when balance is disturbed, the body can make adjustments to help maintain its necessary balance. By simple definition, the basis of all disease is a response to injury. To cure disease, the body must provide a balanced physical response, using a combination of its many inborn healing mechanisms. This propensity for life through the innate healing ability of the body could be demonstrated in every system of the organism; it is built into the intricate design of the DNA of every human being. This phenomenon alone should cause us to bow in adoration of our Creator.

2. Assisted healing

There are times when the body is not able to effectively use its innate healing properties without the intervention of a knowledgeable physician's assistance. Because of severe injury or catastrophic events, such as heart attacks and strokes, the body would not survive without medical assistance. And yet physicians and surgeons are not the only assistants to the healing of your body. Without researchers, we would not be able to apply their invaluable knowledge of the body's "engineering systems" to our healing techniques.

3. Inner healing

Wholeness and balance at the mental and spiritual levels are scientifically proven to affect the capacity of your body to heal physically. Mentally we must have the "mind of Christ" (1 Cor. 2:16), remain positive and hopeful, and constantly rejoice with great feelings of thankfulness. Spiritually we must submit to God's Holy Spirit to reign in every part of our being. And by focusing on eternal life rather than temporal existence, we seek to align ourselves with God and His eternal purposes.

4. Improbable healing

The term *improbable healing* is being defined as documented healings that modern medicine and science cannot account for or explain, nor could they have predicted them. Hospital files across the country contain records of modern-day improbable healings, which cannot be explained or refuted by medical science. Numerous scientific studies initiated by universities and other medical groups show convincingly that patients who received prayer had better recovery rates than those who did not. Some studies indicate that even when the patients did not know they were receiving prayer, they fared better than the others who received no prayer. And the number of studies is growing that indicate positive healing results of prayer, regardless of denomination or proximity to the patient.[1] Of course the Gospels are filled with accounts of improbable healings, which the physicians of the day could not have accomplished. In Jesus' ministry there are accounts of the blind seeing, the lame walking, the deaf hearing, and even the dead being raised. As we bow in deep appreciation and adoration before God, our improbable healing rests in His hands, but many can testify and document that God delighted to surprise them with healing that no one could have predicted.

5. Ultimate healing

As believers, we have the most beautiful part of life to look forward to when life as we know it on earth ends. Ultimate healing is somewhat like graduation day for us—the day God brings a beloved child home to be with Him forever in absolute joy and bliss. While we live our lives on this side of eternity, it is wonderful to meditate on the blessed life that awaits us. Of course for this eternal bliss to be a future reality for us, we must seek to remove our alienation from God and return to alignment with God's design for us in this life. It is necessary to receive forgiveness and to surrender our lives to the Lord Jesus Christ, our great physician. Our eternal reconciliation with God must begin now if it is to be fulfilled after this life is completed.

PERSONAL REFLECTION

_____

_____

_____

_____

Day 29

WAITING ON THE LORD

SCRIPTURE IS FILLED with instruction regarding our need to wait on the Lord, to "be still, and know that I am God" (Ps. 46:10). The Word of God promises that if we seek God, we will find Him (Matt. 7:7), and that if we draw near to Him, He will draw near to us (Jas. 4:8). Our forever relationship with our Creator fills us with hope for the never-ending future. As we wait on God, we must prepare our hearts to commune with Him.

PREPARING OUR HEARTS

As Christians, we need to prepare our minds and hearts to seek God. It is important that we clear away any distractions as we prepare to wait on the Lord. Our focus must be on God as we set aside special times during our day to seek Him in prayer. A time of solitude allows us to bring our whole being to the Lord, to quiet ourselves mentally, and to seek only Him.

In study of God's Word

An important aspect of preparation for waiting on the Lord is the study of God's Word. Scripture is our road map that teaches us how to wait on the Lord, through instruction and through the examples of godly men and women. These examples are filled with wonderful promises of hope for those who seek to know God. Scripture also reveals the grandeur of God and helps us understand our finiteness.

In prayer

There are entire volumes written on prayer. For our purposes, we will highlight a few keys to effective prayer as we wait on the Lord. We must:

- Let our thoughts be conformed to the Word of God.

- Surrender our agendas and cast our needs and concerns on Him.

- Fill our minds with the Word of God to know how to pray.

- Consider our motives in prayer. If we are only asking for things that will gratify us, we have wrong motives.

Prayer is the primary way we grow closer to our Lord. On day 22 we described our Christian lives as a "garden of prayer." However, "no matter how much we desire that relationship...we're never free from obstacles. We must battle our egos, the agendas of families and peers, and what the world tells us about success."[1] Watchful prayer helps us overcome these temptations, because spending time with our Lord keeps us focused on His will.

In hope

Hope is birthed in an attitude of gratitude that causes you to expect joyously, even if you have to wait for the answer. You are assured of the character of God. You can develop a habit of thankfulness toward God and others. Hope puts you into a frame of mind to expect to receive and enjoy in the future. Faith gives substance to hope (Heb. 11:1). While hope is important, it lacks substance until it is rooted in faith. Hope is faith talking aloud, drowning out voices of defeat. Whatever situations we face, we can be filled with hope as we wait on God.[2]

In joy

As our prayer lives progress, we discover what it means to be aligned with God. Our spirits radiate the joy of salvation in all that we think and do, and we won't get tired of doing God's will. As Nehemiah 8:10 says, "For the joy of the Lord is your strength." As such joy grows in us, cultivated by prayer, we experience freedom to give our fears, worries, and problems to God. We then abide in Him, knowing He will provide. Our relationship with God through prayer offers a limitless supply of peace and joy that fills our lives.

In sorrow

In times of pain and sorrow we must learn the strength available to us as we wait on God. While it is not possible to live in this world without suffering, as believers, we have the promise of God to heal our broken hearts (Luke 4:18). He also promises us the comfort of the Holy Spirit (John 14:26), as well as the comfort of fellow Christians (1 Thess. 5:11). And we have the wonderful hope for our future—eternal life with our Savior where there is no more sorrow or suffering.

Waiting on the Lord offers us not only temporal benefits of God's presence in our everyday lives but eternal rewards as well. Not only do we receive peace, joy, and comfort for our earthly lives; we enter into a relationship of profound intimacy with our Creator, deepening our appreciation for Him, which will continue to increase throughout eternity.

PERSONAL REFLECTION

_____

_____

_____

_____

_____

_____

_____

_____

_____

_____

_____

_____

_____

_____

_____

Day 30
The Joy-Filled Life

F OR MANY, *JOY* is a foreign word, one whose significance cannot be appreciated without clear definition. What do you think of when you hear the word *joy*? Perhaps a child who is carefree and secure in parents' love, giggling in delight? Or a quiet romantic dinner with candlelight flickering on the face of the one you love?

C. S. Lewis writes that we discover true joy only when we are looking for something else—which is God. He describes joy as the response or result of the felt sense of God's love in our soul.[1] According to Scripture, God promises a joy-filled life for all who will trust Him. Jesus told His disciples: "These things I have spoken to you, that My joy may remain in you, and that your joy may be full" (John 15:11). He wants us to "en-*joy*" life rather than endure it.

There may be some people who tend to associate joy only with personal comfort, ease, and luxury. But joy is a much deeper and richer experience than that. It is the natural outpouring of our hearts in every relationship and situation of life, as God's presence becomes the central pillar of our lives. When we have a personal relationship with Him, we cannot help but be filled with heaven-filled, glorious joy. Our desire to worship and adore God increases as His presence in our lives increases, which is the source of ultimate joy.[2]

One of the greatest hindrances to living a joy-filled life is looking for joy in all the wrong places. Sometimes we mistake a life full of activities for a life of fulfillment. Some believe that if we search hard enough for that "special someone," we will find joy in the encounter. Unfortunately we do not understand that unless we become the "right" person ourselves, we will continually be disappointed in relationships. The list of choices is endless for those who pursue their goal of a joy-filled life apart from its only true realization—in God alone.

Joy Is a Heart Changed by Knowing God

Until we realize, early or late, that what we seek is not within ourselves, we will not have the joy God intends to give us. Our own pursuits will inevitably lead to despair, frustration, anger, anxiety, and loneliness. Joy is a heart changed by knowing God. It takes our breath away. It is an infinite host of angels singing glory to God. It is the greatest music or words we can ever imagine, and still more. This great joy puts everything else out of our heads and hearts. In turning from earthly things, we find God. And by putting our faith in Him, we are filled with abundant joy.[3]

Inner peace

While knowing God is the prerequisite for living a joy-filled life, it is sadly true that many Christians still lack joy because their minds and hearts are filled with worry and anxiety. True joy depends on total abandonment to God and His sovereignty. As we choose to exercise faith in God, to forgive those who hurt us, and to fill our thoughts with the Word of God, the Spirit of God works in us, producing His supernatural attributes of "love, joy, peace, longsuffering, kindness, goodness, faithfulness, gentleness, self-control" (Gal. 5:22–23).[4] When Christ is fixed in our thoughts, we become recipients of His supernatural joy. We walk with Him in everyday life, at work, and in relationships. He abides in us, and we in Him, and we receive His strength, His love, His peace, and His joy.

Laughter

The laughter of joy releases all the stress and anxiety within us. Psychotherapists have developed laughter therapy as an effective tool in their therapeutic kit. The medical world is using the therapeutic effects of laughter to bring healing to their patients, confirming the truth of the Word of God: "A merry heart does good, like medicine" (Prov. 17:22). God placed within us a valuable, healing emotion expressed through laughter.

Celebration

Too often we use the word *celebrate* for a temporal, trivial event in which we enjoy momentary happiness. A much deeper significance of true celebration is reflected in our worship of God, our Creator and Savior. He wants us to celebrate His love and His gift of salvation by committing our lives to worshipping Him. In our deepest worship we learn to relinquish all to Him.

Living a joy-filled life is based on exalting and worshipping God. Celebrating Him fills us with joy. Praise, love, and enjoyment of God produce in us an everlasting bliss as we struggle in a mean, contemptible world. Humility is essential for the happiness that comes with godly joy. Scripture promises that those who humble themselves in worship of their God will be filled with joy.

> But may all who seek you rejoice and be glad in you;
> may those who long for your saving help always say,

"The LORD is great!"

—PSALM 40:16, NIV

PERSONAL REFLECTION

_____

_____

_____

_____

_____

_____

_____

_____

_____

_____

_____

_____

_____

_____

_____

Conclusion

T HE OLD TESTAMENT hero Enoch knew God in such a way that He walked in His presence daily. Such was the reality of God's presence in Enoch's life that one day God simply "took him" home to be with God forever. (See Genesis 5:24.) Scripture gives many examples of God's manifest presence where God showed Himself in a tangible way: in the burning bush of Moses' desert; in the Ark of the Covenant between the cherubim; as a pillar of fire and cloud protecting the Israelites in the wilderness; as a still, small voice to Elijah; and as the angel of the Lord visiting with Abraham. There are occasions when God still chooses to display His presence in a demonstrative way in the life of a believer, a church, or a nation.

No one is ever the same after such an encounter with the Creator of the universe. An eternal God appears in temporal situations and finite human lives to affect an eternal work in them. Those who have experienced this transforming encounter reflect the love of Christ in their lives. The anointing of His Holy Spirit permeates their attitudes, words, and actions. Yet it is the abiding presence of Christ in our lives that is designed to satisfy our hearts on a daily basis, giving us the companionship and divine love that we crave.

Without cultivating this abiding presence of God in our lives, we will not gain an eternal perspective of life and we will not walk in the fulfillment of personal destiny. Likewise we will not be preparing for a life lived in His presence for all eternity.

Have you noticed that whenever Scripture pulls back the

curtain of eternity and gives us a glimpse of heaven, what we witness is the worship of those who are there? Isaiah saw the seraph worshipping and crying out, "Holy, holy, holy is the LORD of hosts" (Isa. 6:3). And when John the revelator was given wondrous visions of the eternal realm, he saw four living creatures who do not rest day or night, saying: "Holy, holy, holy, Lord God Almighty, Who was and is and is to come!" (Rev. 4:8).

This eternal perspective of unending bliss in the presence of God is the key to everything we have discussed. We were created by an eternal Creator, whose sole desire is to live in communion with His creation—eternally. As we realize the wonders of God's love, we cannot help but bow in humble adoration and be filled with radical gratitude for the gift of life.

This adoring gratitude leads us ever deeper into the heart of God. There we find the ultimate satisfaction our souls crave in intimate relationship with our God. There we discover personal destiny—the divine purpose for which we were born. There we are empowered to face and conquer every difficulty of life. And there we learn to love others as we love ourselves.

Surrender, submission, and selflessness lead to ultimate satisfaction found only in complete abandonment to our Creator. It is a theological and experiential reality that when we bow in subservient worship to God, we are filled with joy. When we get rid of our egos and independence, we find ourselves filled with glorious, abundant peace. We are at peace with ourselves because we have found peace in God. Then we are full of joy because we love God and depend on Him, not ourselves. We must never forget that the fountain of our inner life toward God is receiving the love of God by believing His promises.[1]

One of the main goals of this devotional has been to evoke wonder and awe in your soul by observing the wonders of your

Creator. Our spontaneous response to such divine love is, first of all, gratitude, which we express in our daily lives in a thousand ways. Our next response becomes deep adoration, a giving of worship and honor to the Creator of all.

Worship involves giving something back to God. In a spirit of thankfulness we present Him with a gift for who He is and what He has done, because "The LORD has done great things for us…we are glad" (Ps. 126:3). As we yield our lives to Him, which is His gift to us, we begin to realize the purpose for which we were born—to walk in intimate relationship with God. Because that is our ultimate purpose, we cannot hope to find true satisfaction in any other pursuit. God ordained that we enjoy Him from this life perspective of gratitude for our Creator.

The deepest longing of the human heart is to be known completely and accepted unconditionally. God Himself offers this love relationship to all who seek Him. That profound intimacy is available to all who pursue relationship with their Maker and Redeemer. Can you imagine sharing "secrets" with the Creator Himself? Receiving His counsel and guidance for living an anointed life? All of that and much more becomes a reality in the intimacy of relationship with God through Jesus Christ and by His Spirit.

We can draw very close to God on a personal basis, safely revealing our hearts and minds to Him. God calls us to a life of intimacy. God cries out for us to know Him and beseeches us to live near to Him. He desires for us to understand Him and His inner workings, which have been and will be for eternity, and for us to know our place in those inner workings. Yet we must open ourselves to Him. We have to ask Him to tear down the defensive, protective walls we build to prevent intimacy. Consider the psalmist's cry for intimacy: "Search me, O

God, and know my heart; try me and know my anxieties; and see if there is any wicked way in me, and lead me in the way everlasting" (Ps. 139:23–24).[2]

As we abandon our lives to God and begin to express radical gratitude to our Lord, we won't become victims of material gratification to calm our restlessness and mask our loneliness. We will celebrate our fulfillment in God alone. When we cultivate a lifestyle of radical gratitude, we no longer see ourselves as we once did. We now live in anticipation of His eternal presence. We make all of our decisions based on that premise. We see that our lives on earth are short and soon pass away. But we are with the eternal God forever! When we focus on eternal imaginations, we can understand better how little the possessions and measures of worldly success matter. We can point ourselves toward eternity with Him, working enough to meet the needs of our daily lives without being consumed by the cares of the present day. Instead, we are consumed by our focus on our future with Him—a future that begins now as we are engulfed in His presence.[3]

True satisfaction comes through daily communion with God in an intimate relationship of love. Of course Christ is the key to that intimacy, for we know God through Christ, and we are known to Him through Christ. As we continually surrender our lives to Christ, we can become engulfed in His presence and enter into the fullness of God.

Why not bow your heart before our awesome Creator and ask Him to satisfy your deepest longings with His presence? Jesus declared, "Come to me…and I will give you rest" (Matt. 11:28). He will respond, for He summons you to choose to renounce your independent, self-reliant ways and seek His love. As you embrace the loving heart of your Creator, you will begin to understand and appreciate the wonder that fills all of life.

APPENDIX:

NINE WAYS TO CULTIVATE THE PRESENCE OF GOD IN YOUR LIFE[1]

I LIKE TO MAKE a habit of thinking of as many different ways of cultivating the presence of God in my life as possible. This helps us to develop our love for Him and guards us from failures in life caused by a lack of appreciation for our Creator's love. Consider these nine ways we can overcome this failure and learn to appreciate God.

1. Appreciate nature.

The stars are the majesty of this privileged planet. God's glory is seen in the waters, their tides, and the mathematical intricacies that make nature as gorgeous and as beautiful as it is. The DNA and intricacy of a single cell is evidence of the overwhelming vastness of nature. We can simply look at nature's wonders around us and bow our hearts in worship as we appreciate the beauty of God's creation. Because knowledge enhances appreciation (you can't appreciate what you don't know), I encourage you to read and study an aspect of creation that interests you. You will be amazed at the new level of appreciation you have for your Creator.

2. Appreciate Him with all of your senses.

Scientists understand that the greatest activator of the reticular activating system, the brain's attention center, is *sound*. Because the beauty of music excites and thrills our minds and hearts, worship music is especially effective in helping people experience God. Through the arts or other means that cause a sensory response, we may cultivate an appreciation of God and His presence. Enjoy the fragrances of plant life. Gaze upon the brilliant night sky or the snow-covered mountains. Taste the delicious flavors of your favorite fruits. Feel the cool softness of the grass on your bare feet—and appreciate your Creator.

3. Learn the deeper meaning behind familiar traditions.

Many people have come to know God simply through their religious tradition. Symbolic meaning in religious expressions can cause us to think of the majesty of God and worship Him. However, religious formalities that are not engaged with faith and the Word of God do not bring an intense presence of God into a person's life. This overwhelming presence of God, called the manifest presence of God, can be cultivated in other ways, which we will discuss.

4. Meditate on God's Word.

Scripture teaches that the Word of God is food for our spiritual lives, helping us to cultivate appreciation for God and all of life. The more we study the Word of God and meditate on it, allowing it to fill our minds and hearts, the more we will believe its promises and discover their life-giving power. And as we heed its warnings, we will be spared the consequences of violating the commandments of God.

5. Find a cause that brings glory to Christ.

Adopt a project to help others, and it will cause you to grow in your appreciation of God. For example, work with prisoners; help people recover from homosexuality, drug addiction, domestic abuse, or other problems of society; or help inner-city children. We grow in our love of God and others as we find ways to give to them. Sometimes we call people like these "do-gooders," but they are much more than that. They demonstrate the power of a godly life that is passionate about giving to others.

6. Become a caregiver.

Many physicians are wonderful caregivers. They implement their love of God with their caregiving and make it something that is special. I have physician friends who pray for two or three hours a day before beginning to care for their patients; these doctors have become unbelievably godly people. Sharing God's love with their patients is one of the most wonderful ways they have to enjoy God's presence and live a fulfilled life. In other words, God's presence is felt where there is love shared. This is applicable to all of us. We can show Christ's love through all the various people we care for and show kindness to.

7. Develop enthusiasm for life.

The root meaning of *enthusiasm* is "inspired," which originates from *en theos*—in God. Living a life inspired by God gives us a new purpose for life. Our enthusiasm for life should overwhelm every other difficulty in life, making the difficulties less important. For believers who rest in God's redemption, our enthusiasm for life should be greater than other people's excitement for lesser pursuits. Our satisfaction that results from resting in God's redemptive purpose for our lives should result in great enthusiasm for all of life. In this way God will be most glorified in our lives.

8. Study theology.

In-depth study of the Word of God from a theological perspective is important for all of life. It teaches us how to totally intermingle the Word of God into every area of our lives. Being a theologian is one of the most important pursuits for Christians. It enables us to truly understand why we are here, our purpose, and how to find the meaning of life. For example, when we study the Book of Romans, which has been called the "Constitution of Christianity," we are able to formulate our Christian worldview of life. When we study the Book of Revelation and try to understand the future in God, it enlarges our eternal perspective of life. These kinds of theological studies help us prioritize the mundane activities of the day and focus on the presence of God in our lives.

9. Study the mind of God.

According to Scripture, the mind of God is revealed in every aspect of His magnificent creation. (See Romans 1:20.) Studying the mind of God is overwhelmingly beautiful when you begin to understand, through creation, all that He did so that we could enjoy the gift of life. If we study God's mind, we will truly appreciate what it means to be with Him and to love Him.

Each of these nine avenues for appreciating God will result in having the presence of God in our lives, changing our lives for the better. They will help us understand that, amazingly, our Christian walk is not a religious tradition but a *relationship of appreciation* with a person, Christ Jesus, who died for us to forgive our sins against Him. In our journey toward appreciation for God, it is paramount that we understand we are sinners and need God's redemption for our sin. As we learn to walk with Christ continually in deepening appreciation, our divine relationship will bring an end to our rebellion and indifference. And we will learn to enjoy God from the God-ordained life perspective of appreciation for our Creator, Savior, and friend.

Notes

Day 1

1. John Piper, *Desiring God* (Colorado Springs, CO: Multnomah, 2003), 10, https://www.amazon.com/Desiring-God-Meditations-Christian-Hedonist/dp/0786171901.
2. *Merriam-Webster*, s.v. "appreciate," accessed July 12, 2019, https://www.merriam-webster.com/dictionary/appreciate.
3. *Merriam-Webster*, s.v. "appreciation," accessed July 12, 2019, https://www.merriam-webster.com/dictionary/appreciation.
4. *Merriam-Webster*, s.v. "grateful," accessed July 12, 2019, https://www.merriam-webster.com/dictionary/grateful.

Day 2

1. Ellen Vaughn, *Radical Gratitude* (Grand Rapids, MI: Zondervan, 2005), 46.
2. Cicero, *Pro Plancio*, 80, http://perseus.uchicago.edu/perseus-cgi/citequery3.pl?dbname=LatinAugust2012&getid=1&query=Cic.%20Planc.%2080#80.

Day 3

1. David Jeremiah, *Grace Givers* (Nashville, TN: Integrity Publishers, 2006), https://books.google.com/books?id=AAj9v2oTAvQC&pg.
2. Armand M. Nicholi, Jr., *The Question of God* (New York: Free Press, a Division of Simon & Schuster, 2002), 44–45.
3. Nicholi, *The Question of God*, 44.
4. Nicholi, *The Question of God*, 45.
5. Nicholi, *The Question of God*, 46.
6. Nicholi, *The Question of God*, 47.

7. Nicholi, *The Question of God*, 47.
8. Nicholi, *The Question of God*, 47.
9. Nicholi, *The Question of God*, 47.

Day 6

1. *Merriam-Webster*, s.v. "adore," accessed July 12, 2019, https://www.merriam-webster.com/dictionary/adore.

Day 7

1. Lee Strobel, *The Case for a Creator* (Grand Rapids, MI: Zondervan, 2004), 37–39.
2. Strobel, *The Case for a Creator*, 39.
3. Strobel, *The Case for a Creator*, 41.
4. Strobel, *The Case for a Creator*, 42.
5. Strobel, *The Case for a Creator*, 43.

Day 9

1. Eric L. Knick, "Dear Muslim Reader—Who Do You Say I Am?," International Preterist Association, accessed July 17, 2019, https://www.preterist.org/get-answers/refuting-error/.
2. Knick, "Dear Muslim Reader."

Day 15

1. Blue Letter Bible, s.v. "*'ahab*," accessed July 12, 2019, https://www.blueletterbible.org/lang/lexicon/lexicon.cfm?Strongs=H157&t=KJV.
2. Blue Letter Bible, s.v. "*cowd*," accessed July 12, 2019, https://www.blueletterbible.org/lang/lexicon/lexicon.cfm?Strongs=H5475&t=KJV.

Day 17

1. R. T. Kendall, *Total Forgiveness*, (Lake Mary, FL: Charisma House, 2002), 52.
2. Kendall, *Total Forgiveness*, back cover.

Day 18

1. Blue Letter Bible, s.v. "chen," accessed July 12, 2019, https://www.blueletterbible.org/lang/lexicon/lexicon.cfm?Strongs=H2580&t=KJV; Blue Letter Bible, s.v. "chanan," accessed July 12, 2019, https://www.blueletterbible.org/lang/lexicon/lexicon.cfm?t=kjv&strongs=h2603.

Day 19

1. Andrew R. Fausset, *Fausset's Bible Dictionary*, s.v. "faith," accessed July 12, 2019, https://www.studylight.org/dictionaries/fbd/f/faith.html.

Day 20

1. *Merriam-Webster*, s.v. "surrender," accessed July 12, 2019, https://www.merriam-webster.com/dictionary/surrender.
2. James P. Gills, M.D., *Believe and Rejoice* (Lake Mary, FL: Creation House, 2004), 33.
3. James P. Gills, M.D., *Imaginations*, (Lake Mary, FL: Charisma House, 2004), 168–69.
4. Gills, *Imaginations*, 168–69.

Day 22

1. Gills, *Believe and Rejoice*, 57.
2. Gills, *Rx for Worry: A Thankful Heart*, 44–45.
3. Gills, *Imaginations*, 66.
4. Gills, *Imaginations*, 191.

Day 25

1. Gills, *God's Prescription for Healing*, 80.

Day 26

1. *Merriam-Webster*, s.v. "comfort," accessed July 17, 2019, https://www.merriam-webster.com/dictionary/comfort.
2. *Merriam-Webster*, s.v. "solace," accessed July 17, 2019, https://www.merriam-webster.com/dictionary/solace.

Day 27

1. Richard A. Swenson, *Margin: Restoring Emotional, Physical, Financial, and Time Reserves to Overloaded Lives* (Colorado Springs, CO: Navpress, 2004), 70.
2. Swenson, *Margin*, 70.
3. Swenson, *Margin*, 79–82.
4. Dolores Curran, *Stress and the Healthy Family* (San Francisco: Harper and Row, 1985), 157.
5. James Dobson, *Dr. Dobson Answers Your Questions* (Wheaton, IL: Tyndale, 1982), 27–28.
6. Swenson, *Margin*, 123–128.
7. Don Reisinger, "The Average American Household Has $8,284 in Credit Card Debt," *Fortune*, December 10, 2018, http://fortune.com/2018/12/10/american-household-credit-card-debt/.
8. Swenson, *Margin*, 173.

Day 28

1. R. C. Byrd, "Positive Therapeutic Effects of Intercessory Prayer in a Coronary Care Unit Population," *Southern Medical Journal* 81 (1988): 826–829.

DAY 29

1. "Roadblocks to Prayer," Beacon Light International Baptist Cathedral of Houston, 2006, https://web.archive.org/web/20081011223306/http://beaconlight.org/HTM/pastors_heart/devotion/devotion2.html.
2. Gills, *God's Prescription for Healing*, 99.

DAY 30

1. C. S. Lewis, *Surprised by Joy* (Orlando, FL: Harcourt Brace, 1956).
2. Gills, *Believe and Rejoice*, 6.
3. Gills, *Believe and Rejoice*, 11.
4. Gills, *Imaginations*, 168–69.

CONCLUSION

1. Gills, *Believe and Rejoice*, 45.
2. Gills, *Imaginations*, 82.
3. Gills, *Imaginations*, 45.

APPENDIX

1. The appendix is the author's adaptation of the nine sacred pathways discussed in Gary Thomas, *Sacred Pathways* (Grand Rapids, MI: Zondervan, 2000).

About the Author

James P. Gills, MD, received his medical degree from Duke University Medical Center in 1959. He served his ophthalmology residency at Wilmer Ophthalmological Institute of Johns Hopkins University from 1962 to 1965. Dr. Gills founded the St. Luke's Cataract and Laser Institute in Tarpon Springs, Florida, and has performed more cataract and lens implant surgeries than any other eye surgeon in the world. Since establishing his Florida practice in 1968, he has been firmly committed to embracing new technology and perfecting the latest cataract surgery techniques. In 1974 he became the first eye surgeon in the United States to dedicate his practice to cataract treatment through the use of intraocular lenses. Dr. Gills has been recognized in Florida and throughout the world for his professional accomplishments and personal commitment to helping others. He has been recognized by the readers of *Cataract & Refractive Surgery Today* as one of the top fifty cataract and refractive opinion leaders.

As a world-renowned ophthalmologist, Dr. Gills has received innumerable medical and educational awards and has been listed in *The Best Doctors in America*. As a clinical professor of ophthalmology at the University of South Florida, he was named one of the best ophthalmologists in America in 1996 by ophthalmic academic leaders nationwide. He has served on the board of directors of the American College of Eye Surgeons, the board of visitors at Duke University Medical Center, and the advisory board of Wilmer Ophthalmological Institute at Johns Hopkins University.

While Dr. Gills has many accomplishments and varied interests, his primary focus is to restore physical vision to patients and to bring spiritual enlightenment through his life. Guided by his strong and enduring faith in Jesus Christ, he seeks to encourage and comfort the patients who come to St. Luke's and to share his faith whenever possible. It was through sharing his insights with patients that he initially began writing on Christian topics. An avid student of the Bible for many years, he has authored numerous books on Christian living, with over nine million copies in print. With the exception of the Bible, Dr. Gills' books are perhaps the most widely requested books in the US prison system. They have been supplied to over two thousand prisons and jails, including every death row facility in the nation. In addition, Dr. Gills has published more than 195 medical articles and has authored or coauthored ten medical reference textbooks. Six of those books were best sellers at the American Academy of Ophthalmology annual meetings.

DID YOU ENJOY THIS BOOK?

We at Love Press would be pleased to hear from you if *Journey to Gratitude* has had an effect on your life or the lives of your loved ones.

Send your letters to:
Love Press
P.O. Box 1608
Tarpon Springs, FL 34688-1608